Tell Me What to Eat Before, During, and After Cancer Treatment

Tell Me What to Eat Before, During, and After Cancer Treatment

Nutritional Guidelines for Patients and Their Loved Ones

By Jodi Buckman Weinstein, MS, RD, CSO, CDN

A division of The Career Press, Inc.
Pompton Plains, NJ

TELL ME WHAT TO EAT BEFORE, DURING, AND AFTER CANCER TREATMENT
EDITED BY NICOLE DEFELICE
Cover design by Lucia Rossman/DigiDog Design
Printed in the U.S.A. by Courier

To order this title, please call toll-free 1-800-CAREER-1 (NJ and Canada: 201-848-0310) to order using VISA or MasterCard, or for further information on books from Career Press.

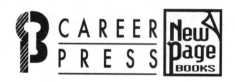

The Career Press, Inc., 220 West Parkway, Unit 12
Pompton Plains, NJ 07444
www.careerpress.com
www.newpagebooks.com

Library of Congress Cataloging-in-Publication Data

Buckman Weinstein, Jodi.

Tell me what to eat before, during, and after cancer treatment : nutritional guidelines for patients and their loved ones / by Jodi Buckman Weinstein.

p. cm.—(Tell me what to eat)

Includes bibliographical references and index.

ISBN 978-1-60163-109-1

ISBN 978-1-60163-727-7 (ebook)

1. Cancer—Nutritional aspects—Popular works 2. Cancer—treatment—Nutritional aspects—Popular works. I. Title.

RC268345.B83 2010

616.99'40654--dc22

2010008941

To my beloved husband and soul mate, Adam. Your pure love, constant support, and organizational skills helped me every step of the way. You brighten my every day and nourish my spirit. To my mom and dad for your support and encouragement to pursue a career as a registered dietitian, and for always teaching me to go for it. And, to my Aunt Midge, forever in my heart, who lost her battle to breast cancer in 2002. Her optimism still inspires me every day.

Publisher's Note

Contents

Introduction

I answered my phone the other day and heard an excited voice on the other end. It was a cancer patient of mine whom I had met six months ago for a nutritional consultation in my office at Mount Sinai Medical Center. She said that she had just completed chemotherapy treatment, survived two brain surgeries, and, surprisingly, felt fabulous! She credits her extraordinarily positive attitude, as well as her post-chemo stamina and overall well-being to eating well throughout her treatments. When I asked her how she was able to maintain such an optimistic outlook, she answered matter-of-factly, "How else can I be?"

This patient exemplifies how good nutrition can lead to a positive attitude during cancer treatment. Through the years as a Registered Dietitian (RD), I have seen that improved nutrition can change the emotional state of many patients, such as a patient with cancer or HIV gaining weight, a patient with diabetes maintaining desirable blood sugar levels, or a patient losing her post-pregnancy weight. I have watched discouraged patients regain a sense of control over their lives by making dietary changes. Being diagnosed with cancer may make you feel somewhat helpless at times, but taking control of your diet may help you feel more in control of your situation.

? How will this book and what I eat help me through my cancer treatment?

This book will guide you through the different side effects of treatments that may change your appetite and nutritional intake. Throughout this book and your treatment, I and other health professionals will discuss your nutrition, nutritional intake, and diet. Good nutrition is a vital part of your cancer diagnosis before, during, and after your treatment. Eating the right amount of food will help you feel better, stay stronger, keep up your energy, maintain your weight, decrease your risk of infection, prevent the breakdown of body tissue, and help you heal as quickly as possible.

Cancer and some of its treatments can cause your appetite to decrease and interfere with eating the right amount of nutrients. Nutrients are classified as *micronutrients*, nutrients you need in small amounts, such as vitamins and minerals, or *macronutrients*, nutrients you need in relatively higher amounts, such as carbohydrates, proteins, fats, and water. The different nutrients that cancer patients need will be discussed in detail in Chapter 2.

This book is designed so that you can read the sections that pertain to you as you need them. You may have started reading this book with no issues that affect your diet, or you may have already experienced some changes in your eating patterns. The book is organized to help you along the way; before, during, and after cancer treatment.

| ? | Is there a "special" diet for cancer? |

No, but there are diet recommendations specific to each side effect. This book will provide you with menu and snack ideas, energy-boosting recipes, and tips for including the right kinds of foods for you at the right times. You may need to continuously modify the way you eat based on the symptom that is preventing you from eating well.

Change the Way You Think About Nutrition

During your treatment, you will need to think about a different kind of nutritious eating. You probably have a general idea of healthy eating guidelines, such as eating fruits and vegetables, whole grain breads and cereals, lean meats and low-fat dairy products, and limiting the amount of fat, sugar, and salt in your diet. Prepare to make some changes in your diet that may seem different from what you previously thought was nutritious eating. Due to the side effects of different treatments, you may need to focus on increasing the amount of calories you eat every day, which may be the opposite of how you ate in the past. Your new diet may include using whole milk instead of skim milk, and your cooking methods might have to be adjusted to include more oil, butter, or margarine. During treatment, you may have to cut back on high-fiber foods, such as fruits and vegetables, to avoid weight loss. It is important to eat whatever works well for you to maintain your weight.

A Few Words About Your Weight

When you are healthy, eating enough is usually not a problem for most people. Most Americans eat adequate amounts of nutrients and few are deficient in any. During cancer treatment, eating may be a challenge. Maintaining your weight is one of the most important things you can do for yourself to help your body heal. Eating is your responsibility, and while the doctors control the chemotherapy that goes into your body, you control the food that goes into your body.

Chapter 1

What You May Expect From Treatment

Diet is estimated to account for approximately 30 percent of all cancers, making diet second only to tobacco as a preventable cause of cancer (source: World Health Organization). In recent years, research has linked overweight and obesity to many types of cancer, as well as linking fruit and vegetable intake and physical activity with having protective effects against some cancers. We can't know exactly what causes anyone's cancer, and there is not one, but many contributing factors to cancer besides diet, such as environment, genetics, and lifestyle factors. However, the statistics show us that we can make changes in our diet and behaviors to decrease the risk of cancer and recurrence.

As you go through treatment, you may need to continuously change your diet based on symptoms. After treatment, you will also need to modify your diet for recovery and survivorship. My goal is that this book helps you feel empowered to make smart choices in your diet and lifestyle—throughout treatment and beyond—to have a healthy future. Focusing on the positive when making any dietary changes before, during, and after treatment. Focus on what *to* eat rather than on what *not to* eat.

For those of you just recently diagnosed with cancer, you are probably feeling anxious and scared about what lies ahead of you. You most likely have met someone who had cancer or heard stories from someone who went through cancer treatment. Your doctor may have already discussed treatment options, which may include surgery, chemotherapy, radiation therapy, hormone therapy, immunotherapy, bone marrow or stem cell transplantation, or a combination of treatments, and most likely informed you of possible side effects from treatment, some mild and some more severe. The good news is that you may, in fact, experience few side effects, which can be controlled with medications and dietary changes. Also, most of the side effects that occur during treatment are temporary and will go away when you finish your course of treatment. I will guide you through all the ways in which you can help yourself through how, what, and when to eat. Dietary changes, along with medications, are the key elements for helping you feel as best as possible during treatment.

The purpose of treating cancer is to kill the cancer cells. Unfortunately, in the process of killing cancer cells, some of your rapidly growing healthy cells, such as bone marrow, hair, and the cells lining the digestive track from the mouth to the anus, can often become damaged. The damage done to these healthy cells causes the physical symptoms to occur, some of which may interfere with your ability to eat well. Additionally, you may have difficulty eating due to your psychological and emotional state. We will discuss more about emotional eating in Chapter 3.

What are the cancer treatments and how can they affect my eating?

Chemotherapy

Chemotherapy is the use of medications that interfere with the steps of the cell cycle involved in the making of your DNA and replication of tumor cells. The goals of chemotherapy are to cure the cancer, control the tumor growth, and improve your comfort and quality of life. Chemotherapy can be used alone or in combination with other treatments, such as surgery or radiation therapy. Chemotherapy is taken by mouth or given by injection into your bloodstream. Your side effects will depend on the chemotherapy medication.

 ## What are some of the common side effects of chemotherapy that may interfere with my ability to eat?

- Loss of appetite
- Sore mouth or throat
- Dry mouth; thick saliva
- Taste and smell changes
- Nausea
- Vomiting
- Diarrhea
- Constipation
- Fatigue
- Depression
- Weight changes (loss or gain)
- Low white blood cell counts, which increases your risk of infection

Detailed diet recommendations for each of these side effects will appear in Chapter 4. You may or may not have all of these side effects from chemotherapy. It is essential that you tell your doctor or nurse if any of these symptoms occur, so that proper medications can be prescribed in a timely manner to prevent any serious consequences, such as severe weight loss, electrolyte abnormalities, or dehydration.

? What are some other side effects of chemotherapy related to nutrition?

Chemotherapy can also cause a decrease in the number of your red blood cells, which is referred to as anemia. Anemia can be caused by chemotherapy, radiation, cancer itself, iron deficiency, folate deficiency, or vitamin B12 deficiency. One of the ways you can help keep your red blood cells working at their peak is by eating well and maintaining your weight. Eating enough calories and protein to prevent weight loss can help your body recover and heal during treatment, help your red blood cells do their job, and help prevent vitamin and mineral deficiencies. If you lose weight, your body will need to use your muscle and other cells in your body, including red blood cells, for energy to live. Focus on eating a high-calorie, high-protein diet if you are losing weight (tips are in Chapter 4). If your red blood cell count becomes too low, your doctor will discuss other ways to medically manage this. Do not supplement with iron, folate, or vitamin B12 unless you have been told you have a known deficiency of these nutrients and your doctor has prescribed them. If you have low levels of iron, there are certain foods that you can eat to help increase your iron intake. Refer to Chapter 4.

Chemotherapy can also cause something called *neutropenia,* and you may hear your health care providers use the words *neutropenic* or *ANC* (which is absolute neutrophil count). If you are *neutropenic* (generally when your ANC drops below 1000–1500/ mm3), you are experiencing a decrease in the number of neutrophils, which are a type of white blood cell that protects you from infections and food-borne illnesses. If you are neutropenic, this means you have a weakened immune system (referred to as *immunosuppressed*) and an increased susceptibility to infection and food-borne illnesses; therefore, you should be following safe food handling practices (see Food Safety Guidelines on page 30). There are no foods that can prevent neutropenia; however, following food safety guidelines will direct you as to what foods are best for you.

? Are there any foods I should avoid during chemotherapy?

For most chemotherapy medications, you do not need to avoid eating any specific foods; however, there are a few that require some dietary changes that your doctor, nurse, or dietitian will discuss with you. For the most part, you will only need to eliminate certain foods based on your symptoms, for example, avoiding fiber for diarrhea, or dry foods for mouth sores.

? How does eating well and maintaining my weight during chemotherapy help me?

Eating the proper amounts of nutrients can help you both psychologically and physically:

- Maintain your energy, stamina, and strength.
- Prevent fatigue.
- Maintain your weight and proper nutrient stores, such as protein and fat (adipose) stores.
- Maintain your emotional well-being.
- Heal and recover quickly.
- Tolerate your treatment as best as possible.

- Increase your response to treatment.
- Improve your quality of life.
- Enhance your daily living activities.

? How can I prepare for the day of chemotherapy treatment?

- Bring snacks or a light meal with you to chemo-therapy that do not need refrigeration (unless you know there is a refrigerator in your facility). Some examples include: a sandwich (like peanut butter and jelly); a bagel; small Ziploc bags of your favorite snacks, such as dried fruits, nuts, trail mix, granola, your favorite cereal, and pretzels; granola bars; crackers; nutrition and energy bars (Power Bars, ClifBars, Balance Bars, Luna Bars, and many others); liquid supplements (Boost Plus or Ensure Plus); and single-serving gelatin, puddings, canned fruits, and peanut butter. Depending on your side effects, you will need to modify what snacks you bring with you based on what you can tolerate. For example, if you are having diarrhea, you should be snacking on bland, low-fat, low-fiber foods such as pretzels or saltines. If you have difficulty chewing or swallowing, you should be snacking on soft or liquid foods, such as pudding, applesauce, gelatin, and yogurt. We will thoroughly review the appropriate foods to eat for each symptom in Chapter 4.

- When packing snacks or liquid supplements, bring enough to last you for traveling to and from the treatment center, as well as for during treatment. If you bring foods that require refrigeration, pack them in a cooler bag.

- If you would like to try nutrition supplements (Ensure Plus or Boost Plus), ask your nurse, doctor, or dietitian if there are samples in your center. There are many brands of nutrition supplements that come in different flavors and forms—liquid and powder—that your center may carry. These supplements help add calories and protein to your diet.

- Do not come to treatment on an empty stomach. Eat breakfast on the day of treatment, and make sure you eat at least one hour before treatments. Have a bowl of cereal with milk and some fruit, or scrambled eggs on toast with a cup of 100-percent fruit juice, such as orange juice.

- Try to get enough rest and sleep at night to reduce the fatigue that is associated with chemotherapy.

- If you are having difficulty preparing food or shopping for yourself, ask friends and family to lend a hand. A trip to the grocery store to stock up on your favorite foods (and foods that you currently tolerate well) will make it so much easier for you to eat well. I have noticed with many of my patients that their food intake declines from simply having a lack of food in the house. If your appetite declines, many people need the reminder of seeing food lying on the counter or in the refrigerator. I often make shopping lists with my patients of their favorite foods, so they can stock up on them for the house. I will provide you with shopping list suggestions in Chapter 6.

- If you do not have anyone to help you with meals, there are programs available that can deliver meals to your home, such as Meals on Wheels. You can also look for community or senior center meals, area churches, and social services. Ask if your center has a social worker available to assist you with resources in your area.

- Aim to eat small, frequent meals and snacks about six to eight times per day instead of three large meals. If you do find that your appetite is better at specific times of the day such as in the morning, eat a bigger portion at that time.

- Check if your cancer center has support groups. Support groups have other patients going through similar experiences. Many patients find it very helpful to talk with other people who are ahead of them in treatment or have completed treatment. Two of my patients in the head and neck cancer support group discussed with each other how they manage dry mouth months after treatment. They expressed to me how valuable it was to know that someone else understood their difficulties and how they found comfort from talking to one another. For more information on support programs, talk to your social worker.

- Avoid heavy, fried, and greasy foods on days you are not feeling well.

- When you are feeling well, go for the foods you enjoy most!

- Drink at least 8 to 10 cups (8 ounces each) of fluid per day.

- Some side effects, such as nausea, go away a few hours after you finish treatment; however, if any symptom persists for longer than that, be sure to immediately tell your doctor or nurse so they can prescribe the appropriate medications to help you. I can't stress enough the importance of immediately alerting your medical team if a symptom arises early stages.

I've had many patients referred to me for a nutrition consultation, and I realized in our meeting that the patient did not mention to the doctor or nurse the start or worsening of a symptom that should have been noted. It may start with something that seems inconsequential and not worth mentioning, such as mild nausea or a small mouth sore, but this is something you must share with your healthcare providers, so they can closely monitor the symptom and immediately give you the right medications to deal with it. I once had a patient referred to me who had significant weight loss within a week. When I reviewed with this patient what he was eating, he told me he had been eating very little because he was vomiting all the time. He told me that even the anti-nausea pill he was taking daily was coming back up. After speaking with his doctor, we changed his anti-nausea medication to a patch that could be placed on his skin and better absorbed. This patient did not realize that he should have told his doctor or nurse that he was vomiting the anti-nausea pill. He thought he was doing all he could by sticking to a minimal diet of only Gatorade, crackers, and rice. He didn't realize that changing his medication to one that he would better absorb would save him a lot of unnecessary agony.

- If you were instructed in the past to follow a special diet for a preexisting disease, such as a cholesterol-lowering, heart-healthy diet, a diabetic meal plan, or a calorie-restricted diet, discuss with your doctor, nurse, or dietitian the ways that you can modify your diet.

Radiation Therapy

Radiation therapy uses radiation to destroy cancer cells and prevent them from growing and multiplying. It is considered a local treatment because it is directed at the part of the body with cancer and only the cells in the area being treated are affected. Both cancerous and healthy cells are affected by the radiation; however, the healthy cells recover more quickly. Your doctor determines your total dose of treatments based on how your healthy cells recover after treatment; therefore, radiation is delivered in small, consecutive doses, usually for two to nine weeks. Radiation is used to treat cancers such as breast, brain, colon, larynx, and prostate cancer, and leukemia and lymphoma. It is commonly used in combination with other forms of cancer treatment, such as surgery and chemotherapy.

Nutritional side effects of radiation therapy

The nutritional side effects you may experience will depend on the area receiving radiation, the size of the area being treated, the total dose of radiation, the number of treatments, and whether you receive it in combination with another form of treatment, such as chemotherapy. Most side effects start around the second or third week of treatment and typically last two to three weeks after therapy ends, although some may last longer (for example, taste changes and dry mouth due to head and neck radiation therapy). If you receive radiation therapy to any part of your gastrointestinal (GI) tract, you are more susceptible to side effects that affect your nutritional status.

You are more at risk for experiencing nutrition-related side effects when the following body parts are treated:

- **Brain, spinal cord:** may cause nausea, vomiting, fatigue, and loss of appetite.
- **Head and neck area (tongue, voice box, tonsils, salivary glands, nasal cavity, pharynx):** may cause sore mouth and throat, dry mouth, thick saliva, difficulty

or painful swallowing, taste and smell changes, fatigue, and loss of appetite.

- **Lung, esophagus, breast:** may cause difficulty swallowing, heartburn, fatigue, and loss of appetite.
- **Abdomen and pelvis (large or small intestine, prostate, cervix, uterus, rectum, or pancreas):** May cause nausea, vomiting, diarrhea, gas, bloating, lactose intolerance, changes in urinary function, fatigue, and loss of appetite.

? What can I do if a side effect develops while receiving radiation therapy?

Similar to the side effects of chemotherapy, you can ask your doctor, nurse, or dietitian whether medications or modifying your diet may help you feel better. Eating well is equally important during radiation therapy as it is during chemotherapy and can help you maintain your strength and your weight, tolerate the side effects of treatment, heal quickly, and decrease your risk of infection.

? How can I prepare for the day of radiation therapy?

Follow the suggestions listed on pages 20–23 for preparing for the day of chemotherapy treatment.

Surgery

Surgery is often the course of treatment for many cancers. Depending on the stage of cancer, your course of treatment can include surgery with chemotherapy and radiation. Surgery is used to remove the cancer cells and any surrounding tissue that may include cancer cells. As with all types of surgeries, your body will go through a process of healing and recovery after surgery, which requires you to eat extra calories and protein. Surgery may cause a temporary decline in your appetite, and constipation from the pain medications and anesthesia. Depending on the location of surgery, you may have difficulty obtaining and digesting the appropriate nutrients. For example, removal of any part of your mouth, esophagus, stomach, small intestine, colon, or rectum may affect your ability to eat and digest essential nutrients. If you have already experienced significant weight loss (5 pounds or more below usual adult body weight), or if you are underweight and weak, you should make an extra effort before surgery to start eating a high-calorie, high-protein diet. It is important to increase your calorie and protein intake a minimum of five to seven days prior to surgery to help improve wound healing, better tolerate the surgery, and have fewer complications afterward. Suggestions for high-calorie, high-protein diets are in Chapter 4.

? What should I eat to help me recover from cancer surgery?

Again, eating well is an important part of your recovery. It's important that you eat enough calories, especially those from protein-rich foods, to help you heal as quickly as possible. Side effects from surgery can be treated with medications, so communicate with your healthcare team as soon as you experience any side effects. Medications along with modifying your diet may help reduce any side effects you experience. See Chapter 4 for ways to manage side effects and ways to add calories and protein to your diet.

Eating and drinking immediately after surgery

Due to the surgical process and anesthesia, the first thing you will be allowed to drink after surgery is clear liquids, such as clear juices, strained citrus juices, strained lemonade, fruit ices, tea, strained chicken or vegetable broth, water, sport drinks, consommé, and plain gelatin. Once your physician determines it is appropriate, you will be allowed to begin pureed, soft, or regular foods (depending on your surgery).

You may be seen by a speech language pathologist at your bedside to test your swallowing function or to provide you with swallowing exercises. You may be told to follow a diet modified in consistency while you are healing, such as a liquid, pureed, chopped (sometimes called "mechanical soft" or "mechanically altered"), or soft diet. While in the hospital, you may ask to speak with a dietitian for more information on your prescribed diet.

? What are some of the side effects from cancer surgery that may affect my eating?

Depending on the location of surgery, the side effects you may experience will vary in degree and length of time. Some of the side effects that may occur following surgery include: difficulty swallowing and chewing, taste changes, dry mouth, sore mouth, heartburn, indigestion, feeling a sense of fullness when eating, fat intolerance, milk intolerance, diarrhea, constipation, high blood sugar levels, gas, cramps, decreased absorption of some nutrients, loss of appetite, and fatigue. Your healthcare team can inform you which side effects are more likely to occur based on the location of your surgery.

Immunotherapy

Immunotherapy, also called biological therapy, enhances the body's immune system to fight the cancer. The main purpose of this treatment is to help stimulate your body's immune system to work harder than usual. It may be used by itself or with another form of treatment to increase its effects. Side effects vary for each person based on the specific treatment provided.

Some side effects of immunotherapy include:

- Fever
- Fatigue
- Muscle aches
- Nausea and vomiting
- Sore mouth
- Dry mouth
- Loss of appetite and weight loss
- Taste changes

Hormonal therapy

Hormonal therapy is used to treat hormone-sensitive cancers, such as prostate, breast, and endometrial cancers. It blocks the cancer cells from receiving the hormones they use to grow. The medications prevent tumor growth by stopping the body from making certain hormones or by changing the way hormones normally work. Side effects for each person vary based on the specific treatment provided.

Some side effects of hormonal therapy include:

- Appetite changes
- Fluid retention
- Weight gain
- Nausea and vomiting

Hematopoietic cell transplantation

Hematopoietic cell transplantation is also referred to as *stem cell transplantation* or *bone marrow transplantation*. The goals of this treatment are to replace defective bone marrow with non-defective marrow. The treatment regimen includes chemotherapy to kill the defective bone marrow stem cells and may include total body irradiation. Depending on the patient's overall health, doses of chemotherapy range from low-dose to high-dose chemotherapy.

These regimens prepare you for the transplant. You may receive cells from yourself, an identical twin, or an unrelated, blood matched donor. Following the transplant, you may experience oral and gastrointestinal side effects. A common side effect that affects eating and nutrition is called graft-versus-host disease (GVHD). A dietitian, nurse, and doctor at your facility will closely monitor you during this time and provide you with medications and nutrition recommendations that are right for you.

? What are some common side effects of cell transplantation?

- Mouth and esophageal sores
- Dry mouth
- Thick, viscous saliva and mucous
- Impaired taste
- Loss of appetite
- Nausea and vomiting

Another result of the transplant is you will be told by your doctor or nurse that you are *neutropenic* and *immunosuppressed*. As stated earlier, *neutropenia* means you have a low neutrophil count, which means your absolute neutrophil count (ANC) is considered low and you are at an increased risk of infection. It is advised that you closely follow food safety precautions to prevent acquiring an infection from food, often referred to as *food poisoning* or *foodborne illness*. Your healthcare team will tell you how long you should be following the immunosuppressed diet guidelines on the following pages. These guidelines should be used along with the food safety guidelines specific to your cancer facility.

Food Safety Guidelines

- Before and after handling all your food, wash your hands thoroughly with a rubbing motion for at least 15 seconds using warm water and soap. Be sure to clean the backs of your hands and around your fingernails. You may use an antibacterial soap, but it is not necessary. Dry your hands with a clean, dry towel or disposable paper towels.

- Be sure to wash your hands thoroughly with soap and water after you touch raw meat, poultry, eggs, and fish and before you touch ready-to-eat foods. If other people are preparing your foods, ask them to please do the same.

- Keep raw meat, fish, and poultry separate from all other foods in the refrigerator, and at the bottom of the refrigerator to prevent them from dripping on other foods. Use a plastic bag around raw meat, fish, and poultry.

- Wash all utensils used on raw meat, fish, or poultry before using them on other foods. Clean your utensils thoroughly by using hot water and dish soap or a dishwasher. When cooking, be sure to use a clean utensil to remove the cooked meat.

- Thoroughly clean your cutting boards between uses with hot, soapy water or a dishwasher. It is easier to keep glass or acrylic cutting boards clean. If you use wooden or plastic cutting boards for raw meat, fish, and poultry, you can put these in the dishwasher. Consider using one cutting board for fruits, vegetables, and other ready-to-eat foods and a separate cutting board for raw meat, poultry, and fish.

- Cook whole meat, ground meat (veal, beef, lamb, pork, goat, game), and ham thoroughly to a minimum of 160 degrees F; poultry, turkey, duck, and goose to a minimum of 180 degrees F; ground chicken and turkey to 165 degrees F; and chicken and turkey breast to 170 degrees F. You should use a meat thermometer and insert it into the middle of the thickest part of the food to test that it is cooked to the proper temperature. The meat should not look pink. To test the accuracy of the thermometer, you can put it into boiling water and make sure it reads 212 degrees F. Keep hot foods at a safe temperature, above 140 degrees F.

- Hot dogs, luncheon meats, cold cuts, and other deli meats must be heated to 165 degrees F before eating.

- Keep your refrigerator at or below 40 degrees F.

- When microwave cooking, rotate the dish a quarter turn once or twice during cooking if there is no turntable. When heating your leftovers, use a lid or vented plastic wrap to cover the food and stir a few times during reheating. Be sure food is cooked to a minimum of 165 degrees F.

- Do not marinate raw meat, poultry, or fish on the counter, but rather in the refrigerator. Also, thaw frozen meat in the refrigerator and not on the counter.

- After eating, refrigerate your leftovers within one hour. Throw away all prepared food after 72 hours (3 days). You can also freeze foods if you don't expect to eat them within two to three days.

- Do not eat raw fish, including sushi or shellfish. Fish with fins should be cooked until it's opaque and flakes easily with a fork. Shrimp, lobster, crayfish, and crab should turn red and the flesh should become pearly opaque. Scallops should turn white or opaque and firm. Cold smoked salmon and lox must be fully cooked. Clams, mussels, and oysters should be cooked until the shells open; however, these may be high-risk foods for people with low white blood counts or those who are immunosuppressed.

- Do not eat raw or undercooked eggs, including soft-boiled eggs, or use cracked eggs. A good way to tell if an egg is cooked well is to make sure that both the yolk and the white are firm. Do not eat foods that contain raw or under-cooked eggs, such as cake batter or cookie dough or salad dressings that contain raw eggs.

- Recipes that contain raw eggs should be cooked to a minimum of 160 degrees F.

- Pasteurized eggs, liquid pasteurized eggs, and powdered egg whites may be used in recipes that will not be cooked.

- Do not eat food past its expiration date. Check the "sell by" and "use by" dates and select the freshest products.

- Wash the top of canned foods before opening and clean the can opener after using.

- When dining outside the home, avoid high-risk foods including anything from salad bars, delis, buffets, potlucks, and street vendors. In fast food restaurants, choose foods that are prepared fresh instead of foods that have been sitting under heat lamps, and use single-serving condiment packets instead of self-serve condiment containers. Avoid raw fruits and vegetables when dining out. Drink only pasteurized fruit juices. If you want to take leftovers home with you, ask the server to bring you a container so you can put the food in yourself rather than having your food transferred in the kitchen. Refrigerate leftovers immediately when you get home.

- Do not eat any food with mold on it, even if you think you can just cut it off. Do not eat any foods that smell strange.

- Do not leave perishable food items in your car.

- Avoid eating unpasteurized milk, cheese, or other dairy products, including Mexican-style soft cheese (queso fresco or queso blanco) made from unpasteurized milk.

- Avoid cold smoked fish, lox, and pickled fish.

- Avoid cheeses with molds and soft cheeses, such as blue-veined cheese, Roquefort, gorgonzola, Stilton, brie, feta, farmer's cheese, Camembert, and sharp cheddar. Avoid cheese containing chili peppers or other uncooked vegetables.

- Avoid raw or undercooked meat, poultry, fish, eggs, unpasteurized egg substitutes, tofu, and tempeh. For tofu that is not pasteurized, you should boil 1-inch cubes for 5 minutes in water or broth before eating or using in a recipe.

- Avoid raw, uncooked sprouts, such as alfalfa, mung beans, radish, and broccoli, as well as raw grains.

- Avoid raw, honeycomb, or non-heat-treated honey. Choose Grade A honey.

- Avoid unpasteurized commercial fruit and vegetable juices.

- Avoid all miso products, unpasteurized beer, and apple cider.

- Avoid raw, uncooked brewer's yeast.

- Avoid unroasted nuts and roasted nuts in their shells. Choose canned or bottled roasted nuts, and shelled and roasted nuts.

- Avoid herbal supplements.

- Avoid salsas found in the refrigerator section of the grocery store; choose shelf-stable salsas.

- Tap water from your home faucet is considered safe as long as your water comes from city water supply or a municipal well serving highly populated areas. Avoid well water from private or small community wells, though it is safe to drink well water if it is tested daily and found to be free of coliforms and Crytosporidium organisms. If your water is not from a city water municipal well supply, you can boil water at home (bring water to rolling boil for one minute), store in the refrigerator, and use within 72 hours. You can also use distilled water (using a steam distillation system), or bottled water labeled as having been treated with one or more of these treatments: reverse osmosis; distillation; or filtered through an absolute 1 micron or smaller filter (certified NSF Standard #53). You can check *www.bottledwater.org* or call 1-800-928-3711 to find out which bottled waters have undergone these processes. If you would like to use a water filter at home, chose filters certified by NSF International (go to *www.NSF.org* or call 1-800-673-8010).

- Wash fruit and vegetables with plain, cold running water without soap or other cleansing products before eating. It is recommended to hold produce under running water in the palms of your clean hands, and gently rub the outside with your fingertips while turning continuously. Be sure to thoroughly wash the stem area and remove all stems. Dry the food with a clean, dry towel or paper towel. You should also wash produce that needs to be peeled, such as bananas, melons, and oranges. For produce with visible dirt on it , or thick, rough skin, such as carrots, cantaloupe, potatoes, and yams, you should purchase a vegetable brush and scrub the produce. You can keep the vegetable brush clean by running it through your dishwasher or rinsing it with boiling water. Rinse the leaves of lettuce and leafy vegetables (spinach, cabbage) individually under running water. It's also best to rinse packaged, pre-washed salads under running water. When dining out, avoid raw fruits and vegetables.

Note: there are some cancer centers and hospitals that recommend avoiding all raw fruits and vegetables except those with thick skins that can be peeled (bananas, citrus fruits, melons) and dried fruits (uncooked) while neutropenic, so follow the guidelines of your center.

*This list was adapted from the Fred Hutchinson Cancer Research Center in Seattle, Washington.

How to Prepare for All Treatments

You can prepare for treatment by asking questions of your healthcare providers and becoming informed about your cancer treatment. Remember to write your questions down and bring them to your appointments. Some patients undergoing treatment have mild or no side effects that interfere with eating, so don't expect the worst.

Become your best advocate and speak up

After working for years in a hospital and outpatient setting, I can firmly say that no health professional can read your mind, so you must learn to speak up and tell your doctors, nurses, and dietitians if any new issues or symptoms arise. You will be asked a list of questions by many health professionals at every treatment and doctor appointment. To prevent the chance of having something that seems insignificant overlooked, it's best to give the most specific details possible to every question asked. This may include you providing some sensitive details about yourself, such as discussing your bowel movements or sharing personal information about financial difficulties. The medical staff at your cancer treatment center can better help you if they have the whole picture in front of them. Throughout this book, I will guide you as to what specific details can change your story. I will show you how to be your own best advocate by speaking up to the medical team about things that may not be asked of you, and by asking questions that you may not have previously thought to ask.

Arm yourself with knowledge

Unlike other medical conditions, cancer can be a visible disease, and depending on its location and treatment, a person's external looks and lifestyle can change during treatment. Only you can truly comprehend what it means to have cancer, and will be the one coping with the side effects that occur. No two people diagnosed with cancer, even those with the same cancer and undergoing the same treatment, will have the exact same experience. That said, I hope you can find some comfort in knowing that other people have had very similar experiences to your own. My goal is to share with you some tried and true tips to help you deal with the side effects of cancer treatment. I hope that reading this book will arm you with the knowledge of what you may expect and how you can handle your diagnosis and treatment.

Chapter 2

Everything You Wanted to Know About Nutrients

Have you ever thought about how your body amazingly digests, absorbs, and utilizes the foods you eat every day? Have you wondered how the nutrients within the foods you eat work to keep you alive and healthy? This chapter will give you some basic nutrition knowledge to help you better understand what exactly you are eating and how the nutrients work within your body to keep you alive. It will provide you with an overview of the six classes of nutrients and discuss how you can adequately obtain the most essential nutrients during cancer treatment. I find that when I help my clients learn the different aspects of the nutrients, they then understand how each nutrient plays its own role in their treatment, and why they may need to put in extra effort to eat well during treatment. By giving you a detailed understanding of these nutrients, you will understand why feeding your body food and liquids is not only crucial for your well-being, but also necessary for survival.

The six classes of nutrients are:

- Carbohydrates
- Lipids (Fats)

- Proteins
- Vitamins
- Minerals
- Water

Among these six nutrients, three of them are considered to be *energy-yielding*, which means they are broken down to give your body energy. The three nutrients that provide energy are carbohydrates, fats, and proteins. The other three nutrients, water, vitamins, and minerals, do not provide energy in the human body; however, they are still vital to life. Many foods have a combination of these nutrients, so when you hear a food described by its nutrient class, such as meat as a protein and pasta as a carbohydrate, it means it is a food rich in those nutrients. For example, in addition to carbohydrate, pasta contains small amounts of fat, protein, vitamins, and minerals. In addition to protein, meat contains water, fat, vitamins, and minerals. Getting enough of these nutrients is very important for people with cancer because cancer itself and some of the treatments for it can greatly affect your appetite, your ability to consume enough food and tolerate certain foods, and your ability to use the nutrients appropriately.

The nutrients you need may differ from another person with cancer. Your doctor, nurse, or dietitian can help you prioritize your nutrient intake based on your condition. Generally speaking, eating a balance of food from all the nutrient classes—carbohydrates, fats, proteins, vitamins, minerals, and water—will help to keep you as healthy as possible to fight cancer.

? What exactly do we mean when we say the word "calorie"?

When you eat carbohydrates, fats, and proteins, the energy released from those foods are measured in calories. The amount of energy a food provides depends on how much carbohydrate, fat, and protein it contains. For example, one gram of carbohydrate and one gram of protein both provide four calories of energy, whereas one gram of fat provides nine calories. This explains why foods with a higher fat content contain more calories than foods with a lower fat content, even though they are the same weight in grams. This also gives you insight into why many of the foods recommended for weight gain are higher in fat because they provide more calories.

Your body requires the energy-yielding nutrients as its fuel for physical activities and metabolism. When describing the importance of eating adequate amounts of all three of the energy-yielding nutrients during treatment, I tell my patients to think about their car. Simply put, if your car does not have fuel (gas), it will not work. By the same token, if your body doesn't get its fuel (calories), it simply will not work. The energy that food provides not only supports your activities of daily living, such as breathing and walking, but it also provides you with the energy necessary to help your fight against cancer.

? What makes me gain or lose weight?

Here's the way weight gain and weight loss work. When you eat food, it first goes to fuel your metabolic and physical activities. Whatever is not used to assist with these activities is stored to be used when energy supplies run low, such as overnight or in-between meals. In short, if you consume more calories than you expend, you will gain weight. Similarly, if you consume fewer calories than you expend, you will lose weight.

An Overview of the Six Classes of Nutrients

Carbohydrates

Carbohydrates are your body's first choice of fuel for energy. If you eat a balance of nutrients at a meal, your body will first use the carbohydrate for energy. They provide fuel for your organs, brain, central nervous system, muscles, physical activity, and everyday tasks. The best sources of carbohydrates are fruits, vegetables, and whole grains. These provide vitamins, minerals, fiber, and *phytochemicals*, which are naturally present in plant foods and help promote overall health.

If you do not get enough carbohydrates, you may experience fatigue, muscle cramps, and poor mental function. If you consume too many carbohydrates, your body stores it in the liver and muscle cells to be used when you are depleted, and anything that is not stored in the liver or muscle is stored as fat.

The two types of carbohydrates are:

- **Simple carbohydrates:** These are carbohydrates that are also referred to as *sugars* and are easily broken down by the body. The better sources of simple carbohydrates are naturally present in foods, such as fructose found in fruits and lactose found in milk. They also contain other important vitamins and minerals. The other forms of sugars often found in processed foods and products with added sugars and syrups, such as soda, candy, and baked products, provide minimal nutrients. We will discuss sugar and cancer in greater detail in Chapter 9.

- **Complex carbohydrates:** These are carbohydrates found in plant-based foods (fruits, vegetables, nuts, seeds, and grains) that typically take the body longer to break down. Starches and fibers are complex carbohydrates. They are commonly found in grain products, whole-wheat bread, whole-grain pasta, brown rice, legumes, and starchy vegetables. When it comes to choosing the best complex carbohydrate grain products, we say "the browner, the better," such as brown rice versus white rice.

A deeper look at dietary fiber

Dietary fiber, also known as "roughage" or bulk, is made up of carbohydrates that your body cannot digest or absorb and which are found in plant foods, such as vegetables, fruits, whole grains, legumes, nuts and seeds. This means that fiber passes through your stomach, intestine, and colon without being digested. High-fiber foods tend to be lower in calories and contain abundant amounts of vitamins and minerals. In the United States, adults consume an average of 15 grams of dietary fiber per day, which is only about half of the recommended daily amount. The National Academy of Sciences Institute of Medicine recommends the following amount of daily fiber for adults:

	Age 50 and younger	**Age 51 and older**
Men	38 grams	30 grams
Women	35 grams	21 grams

The reason fiber is important to understand during cancer treatment is because there may be times you are *told to avoid* or *encouraged to eat* fiber-rich foods based on your symptoms. If you are experiencing nausea, vomiting, diarrhea, or a partial small bowel obstruction, you will need to focus on avoiding high fiber foods and instead focus on eating refined carbohydrates during this time to help with your symptoms and ensure you are eating enough calories. If you are experiencing constipation, you will be encouraged to eat fiber-rich foods as much as possible. More information on fiber will be discussed in Chapter 4.

The two types of fiber are *soluble fiber* and *insoluble fiber*. All plant foods have both types of fiber with varying amounts of each. For example, the insides of most fruits contain soluble fiber and the outside (peel) contains insoluble fiber. The peel of an apple or pear is insoluble fiber while the pulp (inside) of both fruits is mostly soluble fiber.

- **Soluble fiber** dissolves in or absorbs water, helps lower cholesterol and glucose (sugar) levels in your body, and promotes regularity of bowel movements. Soluble fiber helps absorb water which adds bulk and thickens your stool. This type of fiber can be helpful for those with diarrhea. Examples of soluble fiber include oats, oat bran, oatmeal, bananas, apricots, beets, canned fruits, cornflakes, cornbread, grits, boiled rice, carrots, peas, peeled apples and applesauce, oranges, grapefruits, peeled potatoes and yams, turnips, strawberries, acorn and summer squash, barley, papaya, and ground psyllium seeds.

- **Insoluble fiber** does not dissolve in water, helps move food through your gastrointestinal (GI) tract, and promotes regularity of bowel movements. This type of fiber can be helpful for those who are constipated. Examples of insoluble fiber include whole-wheat flour, wheat and corn bran, wheat cereals, rye, brown rice, barley, many vegetables such as dark, leafy vegetables (spinach, kale), the skins of many fruits, flax seeds, beans, peas, lentils, and nuts.

Should I take a fiber supplement?

Most people can eat enough fiber by eating high fiber foods. It is best to obtain fiber from whole foods rather than fiber supplements because whole foods provide vitamins and minerals that fiber supplements do not. Also, research shows that obtaining fiber from whole foods appears to lower your risk of cancer whereas supplements do not. However, for some individuals, fiber supplements may be needed for certain medical conditions, such as irritable bowel syndrome (IBS), high cholesterol, constipation, or diarrhea that is not relieved by dietary changes. Some fiber supplements include Metamucil, Citrucel, and FiberCon, and are sold in the form of wafers, powders, or tablets. Your doctor or dietitian can help you decide if you should use fiber supplements. It is important that you tell your doctor if you start taking fiber supplements because they can interact with certain medications.

Protein

Proteins are made up of two types of amino acids: *essential*, must be obtained from the diet and *non-essential*, body can make on its own. In basic terms, amino acids are the building blocks of protein. Protein plays an integral role in helping the body repair and make new cells and tissue, maintaining the health of your immune system, and assisting with recovery from illness and surgery. Protein is a major component of muscles, organs, and glands and is necessary for growth and development.

During periods of stress and recovery, such as after surgery or during chemotherapy and radiation therapy, your body has increased protein needs. Cancer itself, along with some of the side effects of treatment, can make it difficult to consume adequate protein. Also, cancer causes changes in your protein metabolism, which means if you are losing weight, you are losing lean body (muscle) mass along with fat. During normal metabolism, if you were dieting to lose weight, you tend to lose more fat than muscle mass; however, when you have cancer, your body breaks down muscle and fat at the same time. Basically, this means you will you will need to make an effort to eat additional protein to help with recovery, healing, preventing infections, and maintaining your lean body mass. You must also ensure you are eating sufficient total calories from non-protein sources (carbohydrates and fats) so that your body can use protein efficiently. As stated previously, your body's first source of energy is glucose (sugar), but if your body does not receive enough glucose from the diet during cancer treatment, it will use the protein you eat, along with your muscle and fat, for energy instead. Eating adequate calories along with protein is one of the best things you can do for yourself during treatment to help rebuild red and white blood cells, muscle, and your immune system.

A common secondary diagnosis in cancer patients is a condition called *protein-calorie malnutrition*, or *cancer cachexia*, which is an inadequate intake of all of the energy-yielding nutrients: carbohydrate, fat, and protein. This is caused by factors related to cancer treatment, such as nausea, early satiety, taste changes, and other side effects that interfere with eating well.

Fats

Fats (lipids) consist of fatty acids that may be solid or liquid at room temperature. As stated earlier, fat is an energy-dense nutrient that contains more than twice the calories of carbohydrates or protein. Every gram of fat contains 9 calories, whereas every gram of carbohydrates or protein contains 4 calories. Fats are essential to help insulate your body tissues, store energy, digest and absorb the fat soluble vitamins, and provide a sense of fullness from and palatability in the foods you eat. Consuming dietary fat provides you with essential fatty acids (that you must obtain from the diet and your body cannot make on its own). As previously mentioned, it is important that you eat adequate amounts of non-protein foods, such as fat and carbohydrates, along with adequate amounts of protein foods, so all the macronutrients can do their jobs as efficiently as possible.

? What are the "good" and "bad" fats?

Although fats are important to include as part of a healthy diet, it is important to choose those fats wisely. When counseling my clients, I typically avoid using the words "good" and "bad" when referring to any one food because of the misconception it causes for people. Foods that many people typically consider "bad," such as a piece of cake, can usually be included as a part of a healthy diet, as long as they are consumed in appropriate portion and are accounted for in one's meal plan. So, too, foods that people consider "good" and healthy, such as almonds or whole-wheat pasta, can be consumed in excessively unhealthy amounts. That said, I find it useful to use the terms "good" and "bad" when describing the types of dietary fats.

The "good" fats are the unsaturated fats: *polyunsaturated fatty acids* (PUFA) and *monounsaturated fatty acids* (MUFA). These are considered the "good" fats because they help keep your cholesterol level down and reduce cholesterol deposits in artery walls. According to the American Heart Association, you should limit the amount of *saturated fats* and *trans fats* (the "bad" fats) in your diet because these fats are the main dietary factors raising your blood cholesterol level and increasing your risk for cardiovascular disease, heart attack, and stroke. Note: If you are losing weight during cancer treatment, you can temporarily choose to eat any fats ("good" or "bad") to maintain your weight.

The different fats

- **Saturated fats:** Food sources include mostly animal sources and some plant oils: whole milk, cream, ice cream, butter, lard, meats, whole-milk cheeses, palm, palm kernel, and coconut oils, and cocoa butter.
- **Trans fatty acids:** These fats are actually naturally unsaturated; however, they undergo a chemical process called "hydrogenation" (this adds hydrogen, which saturates the fat), which makes it behave more

like a saturated fat. I'm sure you are well aware of these fats from the recent buzz in the media and emphasis on a "trans fat ban" for restaurants and foods. Many food products on the market contain hydrogenated or partially hydrogenated vegetable oils; recently however, food companies and restaurants are removing hydrogenated fats from products ("trans fat free") because of all the research showing their harmful effects. Some examples of foods that contain trans-fats include cookies, crackers, cakes, french fries, fried onion rings, and doughnuts.

- **Polyunsaturated fatty acids (PUFA) and Monounsaturated fatty acids (MUFA):** MUFA food sources include: olive, canola, and peanut oils; olives; peanut butter; nuts; and avocados. The two types of essential PUFAs are *omega-3* and *omega-6* fatty acids, but you should focus on increasing your intake of omega-3 and decreasing your intake of omega-6. Omega-3 sources are listed on page 47.

? Are Omega-3s important during cancer treatment?

Omega-3 fatty acids are known for their anti-inflammatory effects, and including foods rich in omega-3 fatty acids is associated with preventing heart disease, a lower incidence of some cancers (breast, prostate, and colon), and may have benefits for cancer patients during treatment. The three types of omega-3 fatty acids are alpha-linolenic (ALA), eicosaentaenoic acid (EPA), and docosahexaenoic (DHA).

Some studies suggest that omega-3s may help improve *cancer cachexia* (a condition associated with cancer that includes weight loss, poor appetite, and muscle wasting), improve quality of life, and possibly improve the effects of some cancer treatments. Although the data is mixed on whether omega-3s benefits those with cancer cachexia, some research suggests that about 2,000 mg of EPA per day may help. Because research is still needed in this area, it is recommended that you include omega-3–rich foods as part of your overall diet and use caution with supplements. If you wish to take an omega-3 supplement, please discuss this with your doctor as there are times when it may be harmful. To help incorporate more omega-3s into your diet, try eating a variety of omega-3 fatty fish (such as salmon, tuna, sardines, mackerel, herring, trout, halibut, oysters, and so on) at least two times per week, and choosing plant sources of omega-3 whenever possible. Besides fish, other foods rich in omega-3 include soybean, canola, hemp, rapeseed, cod, liver, walnut, and flaxseed oils; avocados; walnuts; flaxseeds; pumpkin seeds; soybeans; soy foods; and some vegetables. Also, many food companies are fortifying foods such as milk, eggs, cheese, yogurt, butter spreads, and cereals with omega-3s. For those of you who are not fish eaters, flaxseeds are an excellent plant alternative to eating fish. Flaxseeds not only contain significant amounts of omega-3s, but they also provide fiber! One tablespoon provides 3.5 grams of fiber, which can help you reach your goal of 25–35 grams of fiber per day. You can add 1–2 tablespoons of ground flaxseeds to smoothies, yogurt, cereal, oatmeal, salads, frozen yogurt, desserts, chopped fruit, soups, and stews.

Water

Water makes up about 60 to 70 percent of your body weight and is an essential nutrient responsible for a number of important functions in your body. It helps move nutrients between cells and organs, regulates your body temperature, and maintains your hydration status and electrolyte balance. Consuming adequate fluids and water during treatment is extremely important to prevent dehydration, especially if you are experiencing vomiting or diarrhea. Because these side effects can cause a loss of fluids and electrolytes, you must pay attention to replacing fluids and electrolytes (sodium and potassium). If you are vomiting or have diarrhea, you will find suggestions for the best liquids for each symptom in Chapter 4. In general, you should be drinking at least 8–10 (8 ounce) cups of water or clear liquids per day. This amount may change, depending on your treatment. You can reach your daily amount by drinking water, seltzer, club soda, clear fruit juices (such as apple or cranberry) and drinks, sports drinks, clear soups and broths, popsicles, fruit ices, gelatin, soda, and tea. It is best to drink liquids after or between meals to help optimize both your fluid and calorie intake. Some signs of dehydration are thirst, decreased urination, fatigue, lightheadedness, and dry mouth and lips. If you are unable to drink enough fluids, your doctor may prescribe intravenous fluids.

Vitamins and minerals

Vitamins and minerals are among the six classes of nutrients that are referred to as the *micronutrients,* meaning nutrients you need in small amounts. Vitamins and minerals function as hormones, coenzymes, and antioxidants, and are required for cell and tissue growth. They play a crucial role in metabolism and help with the body's use of calories, yet do not provide calories. This area of nutrition is one of the most questioned areas when it comes to cancer patients. Countless numbers of my patients continuously ask me, "Are there any vitamins that I should be taking during cancer treatment that can help me?" Vitamin and mineral supplementation during cancer treatment remains a controversial topic. Many cancer patients look to vitamin and mineral supplements as a way to boost their immune system and help prevent the side effects of treatment. While some supplements may sound intriguing, it is important to note that boosting your immune system with a supplement may actually cause harm and prevent your cancer treatment from working effectively. High doses of vitamins and minerals, such as the antioxidants—vitamins A, C, and E, and selenium—may reduce the effectiveness of chemotherapy and radiation therapy because they could repair the damage done to cancer cells by the treatment. Also, some chemotherapy agents can interact with vitamin and mineral supplements, thereby causing the medication to be less effective. Although there is no clear-cut answer as to whether dietary supplements are harmful, we err on the side of caution and say to avoid the use of any supplements during treatment that contain more than 100 percent of the daily value for antioxidants. If you are taking any vitamin or mineral supplements, please discuss this with your doctor.

We know that there is not a vitamin or mineral that can cure cancer; however, what we do know is that that eating a healthy, balanced diet, exercising, avoiding tobacco, and drinking alcohol in moderation (or none at all), can help lower your risk of many diseases, including cancer. Also, eating a balanced diet that contains adequate macronutrients—carbohydrates, protein, and fats—usually means that you are getting 100 percent of the recommended daily vitamin and mineral needs. Because cancer treatment may interfere with eating a balanced diet, your doctor or dietitian may suggest taking a daily multivitamin and mineral supplement if it appears that you are not eating a balanced diet.

? Can you explain exactly what antioxidants are and if they can help me?

Antioxidants are substances that can prevent or slow the oxidative damage caused by *free radicals*. Free radicals are unstable molecules that are natural by-products of normal cell processes. Exposure to environmental factors, such as tobacco and radiation, can lead to the formation of free radicals. Antioxidants are referred to as "free radical scavengers" that repair or prevent damage done by the free radicals. Free radical damage may lead to cancer, and antioxidants are known to interact with these free radicals and prevent the damage they might cause. Studies suggest that those who include fruits and vegetables, which are full of antioxidants, in their diets on a daily basis may have a lower risk of some cancers. The use of antioxidant supplements has not been proven effective at reducing cancer risk; therefore, health experts agree that the best way to get antioxidants is through foods rather than supplements. If you would like to include antioxidants in your diet, aim to eat a variety of different colored fruits and vegetables. Fruits and vegetables are the richest sources of antioxidants, and the more variety of colors you eat, the more variety of *phytonutrients* (plant nutrients) and antioxidants you will get. Grains, nuts, and some meat, poultry, and fish also contain antioxidants. Examples of antioxidants include lycopene, lutein, vitamin C (ascorbic acid), vitamin E (alpha-tocopherol), vitamin A (beta carotene), and selenium. As stated earlier, if you are undergoing cancer treatment, high doses of antioxidant supplements during cancer treatment is *not* recommended, as they may cause more harm than good. Also, if you are losing weight during treatment, it is not the best time to focus on eating a diet rich in antioxidants because most of these foods contain a lot of fiber and are low-calorie.

? I've taken herbal supplements, such as echinacea, in the past. Can I continue taking them or do they interfere with my cancer treatment?

Surveys show that many Americans use herbal supplements to help treat or improve a medical condition or disease. Herbs fall under the umbrella term of Complementary and Alternative Medicine (CAM), which are remedies often used in place of or in addition to conventional therapy. You will often see herbal remedies in the form of pills, liquids, teas, and ointments. The problem with taking herbal supplements during cancer treatment is that many herbs can interfere with cancer treatment, causing harm and making your treatment less effective. Not only can herbal supplements interfere with cancer treatment, they may also interact with other medications you are taking, making them less effective and not able to do their job properly. If you are taking herbal supplements, be sure to inform your doctor or nurse. Some complementary therapies that may help you with coping through treatment and reduce anxiety and stress include reflexology, biofeedback, meditation and massage, music therapy, yoga and t'ai chi, and acupuncture.

Dietary Supplements and Herbal Remedies

Currently, the U.S. Food and Drug Administration (FDA) does not require manufacturers to print possible side effects on their labels, and there are no laws controlling the safety, content, and quality of these supplements. Because there are no federal standards on these supplements, misbranding and deception are a concern, and you should practice safety precautions by talking to your healthcare team about any supplements you are considering using. Reliable Websites to search for information on CAM are listed in Chapter 8.

How to Obtain Adequate Nutrients

If you are having difficulty swallowing, chewing, eating, or drinking enough during treatment, there are other ways you can obtain adequate nutrients besides using your mouth. The different feeding modalities are referred to as *artificial nutrition support*. Working with cancer patients, I have seen fear and panic set in when the topic of a feeding tube is discussed, sometimes more so than the discussion of any other side effect of treatment. After many lengthy conversations with patients, I know that most people have misconceptions when it comes to the topic of feeding tubes. In many people's minds, it is often associated with end-of-life care, the elderly population, helplessness, and loss of dignity. A feeding tube is actually the opposite of helplessness and does not imply end-of-life care. It is usually one of the most helpful things you can do for yourself during treatment if you are unable to eat enough. My hope is that you read this explanation with comfort and not trepidation, knowing that nutritional support can be extremely helpful during your rough times, can relieve a lot of unnecessary stress during treatment, and may allow you to maintain your independence and dignity. Also, for most people, nutritional support is only used as a temporary solution.

Let's review all the options available for obtaining nutrients. They include: via mouth, via a feeding tube, or via intravenous nutrition, referred to as total parenteral nutrition (TPN). If you are losing weight and having difficulty eating enough food or drinking enough liquids by mouth, the first course of action is to help give you dietary suggestions to increase your calories, protein, and fluids using your mouth (see Chapter 4). If your treatment course makes it too strenuous for you to eat, makes swallowing or chewing extremely challenging, and you continue to suffer from significant weight loss despite dietary modifications, you may need to have a feeding tube placed into your stomach or intestines. A feeding tube can be placed through your nose into your stomach for temporary nutrition support. If you need it for longer than a month, it can be placed directly into your stomach (called a gastrostomy tube, or percutaneous endoscopic gastrostomy [PEG]). It can also be placed in your intestines (called a jejunostomy tube or percutaneous endoscopic jejunostomy [PEJ]).

A feeding tube may be used as a sole source of nutrition or to supplement what you are eating by mouth. Tube feedings can be given at home or at work, so you may be able to continue with your daily routine. The surgery used to place a feeding tube is simple (typically lasting about 20 minutes), can be done as an outpatient procedure, and has little risk and discomfort associated with it. The tube is not painful, cannot be seen underneath clothing, and can be taped to your stomach when not in use. Once the tube is placed, you will feed yourself commercial liquid formulas that can provide 100 percent of your calorie, protein, vitamin, mineral and fluid needs. There are dozens of commercial formulas on the market, and a dietitian will determine which formula is best for you, and how much you need to give yourself daily. These formulas contain the correct proportion of carbohydrates, protein, fat, vitamins, and minerals necessary for survival, as well as the appropriate consistency and thickness to prevent clogging of the tube. I recommend avoiding using non-commercial formulas (homemade blended formulas) because of the risk of clogging the tube, and the difficulty ensuring that you are getting the right proportion of all the nutrients you need.

Feedings can be given as meals, just as you would eat normal meals by mouth, such as breakfast, lunch, dinner, and snacks. They can also be provided as overnight feeds while you sleep, which allows you to have a better appetite during the day if you are still eating by mouth. Your dietitian, nurse, or doctor will review these methods with you and instruct you exactly how to feed yourself.

Most people with feeding tubes can still eat by mouth and will be encouraged to do so, if possible. Even eating or drinking small amounts per day helps to keep your swallowing function intact. A speech language pathologist (SLP) can provide you with suggestions for swallowing exercises if your swallowing function becomes compromised as a result of surgery, chemotherapy, or radiation to the head and neck region. Ask your doctor to refer you to a speech pathologist if one is not available in your cancer center.

Another nutrition support option is *total parenteral nutrition* (TPN), which is nutrition given through a central vein and is commonly used for those with digestive problems who are unable to tolerate feeding through their gastrointestinal tract as a result of surgery or treatment; for those who have blockages within their intestines; or for those with severe vomiting or diarrhea. Similar to a feeding tube, this method may also be used as a supplement to eating by mouth or as a sole source of nutrition. Unlike tube feedings, TPN does not rely upon normal digestion and absorption of nutrients; therefore, it is reserved for those who cannot properly absorb nutrients.

It may take some time getting used to a new feeding regimen, but you will eventually become more adjusted to it. You may want to hear about how others with feeding tubes or TPN are coping with these feeding methods. Ask your healthcare team if they can connect you to someone else in the same boat as you. There is also a resource for those living with home IV and tube feedings called The Oley Foundation, *www.oley.org*, which provides useful information and psycho-social support to patients and caregivers.

Chapter 3

Pretreatment Diet Planning

Now that you've learned about the different types of treatments and their side effects, and you understand how the different nutrients play a role in your treatment, you may be thinking to yourself, *How am I going to feel during my treatment?* There is no way to know exactly how you will feel because no two people experience the same things. During normal life situations, many people avoid being "me" people and have a hard time focusing all their energy on themselves. This is a time in your life when you will need to focus on yourself more than usual. When help is offered, you should accept it. This may sound obvious, but I have watched people undergoing treatment become frustrated with themselves and their loved ones when they need physical assistance from others, such as grocery shopping or cooking. For many of you, this is and will be the hardest thing you will ever have to endure, and you may find yourself surprised by new emotions you never had before, upset by having to rely on others, and frustrated by the unsolicited attention you receive. Finding ways to stay relaxed and keep as positive as possible can help you feel more in control of your situation.

? What is emotional eating?

In general, we know that there is an emotional component to eating for everyone. There are different ways that people use food to cope with stress, sadness, and anxiety. When faced with a stressful situation, there is the person who tends to eat (sometimes excessively), and, on the other hand, there is the person who tends to avoid eating. To illustrate this example of emotional eating, I often tell my clients to think of this scenario: imagine that you have a big deadline at work approaching in a few hours. When faced with this pressured feeling, do you tend to "pick" at snacks and food while working, or are you not in the mood to eat and too distracted to think about eating? The answer to this question can help you understand how your state of mind can affect your eating, and may also give you insight into your own tendencies. Many people do not realize what they subconsciously do when they are anxious, such as using food to cope with their issues.

When it comes to cancer, many people experience a loss of appetite, which may be caused by the cancer itself, fears and worries, or the course of treatment. Even if you were someone who typically grabbed for food in times of stress, you may be surprised to see the opposite occur during your treatment; you may see yourself avoiding food. You may experience worse days than others, and may not feel like eating at all because of feeling sick. This book will give you suggestions for dealing with you appetite and eating issues.

? What can I do if my emotions affect my appetite?

(Answered by Alison Snow, LCSW, OSW-C Oncology Social Worker, The Tisch Cancer Institute):

It is normal during treatment to feel sad, angry, afraid, or frustrated, and these feelings may affect your appetite. There may be periods of time during and after treatment that you feel too sad to eat, sleep, or partake in activities. However, if your sadness becomes overwhelming and you feel depressed, you should seek professional guidance. According to the Diagnostic and Statistical manual of Mental Disorders (DSM-IV), some signs of depression to be aware of include:

- Constant sadness
- Irritability
- Hopelessness
- Trouble sleeping
- Low energy or fatigue
- Feeling worthless or guilty for no reason
- Significant weight change
- Difficulty concentrating
- Loss of interest in favorite activities

Tell your healthcare professional if you're experiencing any of these symptoms. It is important to pay attention to your emotions and relay your feelings to your treatment team. There are professionals who are available to speak with you before, during, and after treatment. A social worker is usually available to speak with you or your family at most cancer centers. Ask your oncology nurse or doctor for a referral if a social worker is not readily available.

There are many resources available to you during your treatment. There are usually support groups available in your community. If you have difficulty finding a group that meets your needs, there are many groups available that are Web-based and phone-based.

- Cancer Hope Network: *www.cancerhopenetwork.org* (877) HOPE-NET
- Imerman Angels: *www.imermanangels.org* (312) 274-5529

- Cancer Care's Website: *www.cancercare.org*
  (800) 813-HOPE
- The Wellness Community: *www.wellnesscommunity.org*
  (888) 793- WELL
- The American Cancer Society: *www.cancer.org*
  (800) ACS-2345
- Association of Cancer Online Resources: *http://list-serve.acor.org*
- AMC Cancer Information & Counseling Line:
  www.amc.org (800)525-3777
- American Psychosocial Oncology Society (APOS):
  www.apos-society.org (1-866-276-7443)

? How can I prepare for cancer treatment in a way that will help my nutritional status?

If you have not experienced weight loss, focus on eating a healthy, well-balanced diet to prepare your body for your cancer treatment. This includes eating lean protein sources, such as legumes (beans), fish, chicken, and eggs, as well as plenty of vegetables, fruits, and whole grains to give your body healthy nutrients to assist with healing. If you have experienced weight loss, you can begin to incorporate a diet that is higher in calories and protein (see Chapter 4).

For those of you who have not lost weight, you can start eating healthy right now.

- If you were not a breakfast eater in the past, now is the time to change that! Eating breakfast helps jump-start your metabolism, and is often a time when people feel the hungriest. I notice that many of my clients enjoy breakfast foods the most when they are not feeling so well. You can try a few scrambled or hard-boiled eggs to give you protein, along with a few slices of bread, toast, or whole grain pancakes or waffles to give you carbohydrates. For those who enjoy cereal, have a bowl of oatmeal or whole-grain cereal topped with some fresh or frozen berries or other fruit to boost your morning vitamin intake. If you're a nut person, add some walnuts or almonds, which provide you with heart-healthy fats. As for your beverage, have a cup of 100-percent fruit or vegetable juice, or a cup of skim or 1% milk.

- Aim to eat a healthy and balanced lunch every day that includes protein, carbohydrates, and fats. Some ideas for lunch are a tuna, chicken, or turkey sandwich, or peanut butter and jelly sandwich on whole wheat bread. Try to include different colored fruits and vegetables in your lunch (chopped vegetables such as baby carrots, celery, cauliflower, broccoli; red, yellow, or green peppers; and fruits such as apples, oranges, or berries). If you enjoy milk, have a cup with your lunch.

- Don't skimp on your dinner. Eating dinner is important to help keep you satiated through the night. You should try to eat a balanced meal that includes lean protein, whole grains, vegetables, and fruits. Eat a pre-bedtime snack if you are hungry later in the night. Be sure to have a snack at least one to two hours before you lie down to sleep to prevent the possibility of reflux.

- If you were not a "grazer" or "nibbler" in the past, now is the time to change that. Instead of eating three large meals, aim to eat five to six "mini meals" and snacks per day. You can start by trying to add a mid-morning and mid-afternoon snack to maximize your daily nutrient intake. Learning how to eat small, frequent snacks is good for everyone, not just those with cancer. It helps keep your metabolism at its peak and helps keep your energy levels stable throughout the day. Write down some of your favorite snacks and give this list to your family or friends so they know how to shop for you, if you need them to do this during treatment. You can also buy some of these snacks in advance so you feel prepared.

Before your treatment begins, you can start planning ahead to prepare for how you will eat during treatment. Here are a few suggestions:

- Don't get too caught up in eating healthy foods if your appetite begins to decline. Eat whatever makes you feel comforted and keeps your weight stable. You can resume healthy eating after treatment.

- Discuss with your family and friends that your appetite may decline during treatment and that you may need them to help you with food shopping and preparing meals.

- Focus on comfort foods. Think about the types of foods you prefer when you feel sick with the flu. Stock up on these foods before treatment. Bland foods, such as oatmeal, plain pasta, farina, applesauce, yogurt, soup, crackers, white bread for toast, and Gatorade are all good possibilities.

- Keep a wide variety of the snack foods readily available at home and at work to eat when you are hungry. You can even cook food or soup in advance and freeze small portions. Seeing food around your house can help remind you to eat when your appetite is lacking. See snack food ideas listed in Chapter 5.

- Prepare yourself for the possibility that you may be eating very differently than you normally have in the past. Foods that you once you loved may not appeal to you during treatment. Foods that you may not have cared for in the past may be new foods that give you comfort during treatment. Try to keep an open mind about trying new foods and listening to your cravings. I've had patients tell me that they didn't particularly like salty foods in the past, yet during treatment, they craved it. Or, I've had patients say they never enjoyed sweets, but then find themselves enjoying sweets during treatment. Avoid eating foods that you love if you are feeling nauseated or very sick, as this can cause an aversion to that food.

• Don't be surprised if you feel that sometimes you are forcing yourself to eat. If your appetite declines, remember that this typically is only temporary during treatment, and should pick up again afterward. Think of food as medicine that will help you get through treatment. The same way you take your medications as prescribed by your physician, you should think of food and liquids as something prescribed to you that you must consume to help you get through treatment.

• Talk with your doctor, nurse, or dietitian about any concerns you have about your nutritional status.

? Can I exercise during treatment?

As long as you check with your doctor for clearance, health experts generally recommend engaging in moderate exercise during treatment and afterward. For all individuals, exercise is known for its beneficial effects on self-esteem, self-image, mood, cardiovascular function, muscle strength, and can help energy levels. Some studies have suggested that cancer patients who engage in several hours per week of moderate physical activity may have fewer side effects from treatment, including fatigue. Fatigue will be discussed further in Chapter 4.

Refocus Your View of Healthy Eating

The following chapter will outline the common side effects of cancer treatment that may impact your nutritional intake. As mentioned before, remember that this is not the time in your life when eating a perfectly healthy diet is necessary. I consider the perfect diet for you a combination of eating any foods that you enjoy and tolerate during treatment that help maintain your weight. Maintaining your weight is one of the most important things you can try to control through treatment with underestimated beneficial effects. The research indicates that weight loss during treatment is associated with more treatment breaks, decreased response to treatment, increased hospital stays, lower quality of life, and the need for lower doses of treatment (Von Meyenfeldt, Maarten, 2005).

Chapter 4

Managing Your Diet During Treatment

This chapter may be useful to read before treatment, but will likely take on a new meaning when you are going through treatment. I outline the common symptoms that are associated with cancer treatments, and my hope is that you use this chapter as a "go-to" reference to flip through for any symptom that may arise throughout treatment. Whether you have none or a few of these symptoms, you can choose to read through all of them or just the ones that pertain to you. The way you eat during treatment will be based on what symptom arises. It's important that you pay close attention to your side effects and modify your diet using the tips in this chapter to help prevent any side effect from becoming severe and causing drastic weight loss or malnutrition. As I tell my patients when I first meet them, we are not laying out all the possible side effects to scare you; rather, we are prepping you for what might be ahead of you. My patients often tell me they appreciated knowing ahead of time some of the things to expect instead of being surprised. You can ask your healthcare team to let you know which of these side effects are more common for your specific treatment and medications.

The first time I meet someone with cancer to review some of the possible side effects that can change their eating patterns, I see that for most people, it is difficult to conceive that they would ever lose their appetite, avoid eating, or possibly experience severe weight loss. For most people, gaining weight has been a problem they've dealt with in the past.

I cannot stress to you enough the importance of doing everything possible within your power to take in the nutrients you need to battle cancer and prevent weight loss. I suggest that if you are reading this chapter before treatment and before any symptom presents itself, you should read it again when you need it.

Similar to physicians, who have a whole bag of tricks for treating illnesses, dietitians possess similar tools for working around side effects and helping you meet your nutritional goals. After reviewing some of these tricks with my patients, I can tell you that I've had dozens tell me that they believed they were doing the right things to help themselves, yet actually they were not. And not only patients, when caregivers and loved ones hear some of the diet tips outlined, they too are often surprised to hear that some of their efforts, while they may be thoughtful and generous, were not necessarily the best thing for the patient. You should feel comfortable knowing that no matter what the side effect, you will be able to make small changes to get the nutrition you need to endure treatment. Even one simple recommendation from the following lists can help you tremendously. There really is a whole bag of tricks! Keep reading, and you will see for yourself.

Common Side Effects of Cancer Treatment

Loss of appetite

Losing your appetite is often described to me as one of the most surprising side effects that a patient experiences. Again, for most people, it is difficult to imagine that they could lose their appetite, and even more so, to lose their appetite for foods that they've loved their whole life. The emotional aspect and connection to food is innate and starts as early as infancy; therefore, when you feel disconnected to food, you and your loved ones usually notice it immediately. If you begin to notice a disinterest in food and the act of eating, it can be very frustrating. As many clients have told me, it is upsetting when something that once brought you so much joy and reminded you of fond memories is now something that can feel more like a chore. Having no interest in a food that used to bring you comfort can feel unfamiliar and upsetting. Remember that this is not permanent; it will pass, and there are many things you can do to help maximize your appetite. For most, your normal appetite will resume after treatment.

Some of the reasons you may experience a loss of appetite (the medical term for loss of appetite is anorexia, although do not confuse this with *anorexia nervosa*, which is an eating disorder) include the cancer treatment itself, stress, depression, and anxiety. This is one of the most common side effects of chemotherapy treatment. While a lack of appetite can cause emotional distress, it can also cause physical distress. As expected, a loss of appetite typically leads to weight loss as a result of eating less overall calories per day. As described earlier in this book, losing weight can cause fatigue, prevent proper recovery and healing, and cause breaks in your treatment. The list of recommendations is expansive because among all of them, hopefully, you will be able to make small modifications that will make big changes.

The following suggestions are ways to improve your appetite, whereas more specific ways to increase calories and protein will be listed in the section on weight loss. If your appetite is poor for an extended amount of time and the dietary suggestions outlined below are not preventing weight loss, you can ask your doctor if appetite-stimulating medications such as Megace or Marinol are appropriate for you.

Ways to improve your appetite

- Eat small, frequent meals and snacks instead of three large, main meals. Begin with five to six mini-meals throughout the day. For those who are going through treatment and losing weight or suffering from poor appetite, increasing this to six to eight times a day will make these side effects more manageable. This helps to maximize your caloric intake and metabolism. Be sure not to miss the opportunity to eat when you feel hungry, and eat whatever your mood and cravings are telling you to eat.

- A lot of people feel the hungriest in the morning at breakfast time, and this is because you are literally "breaking your fast" from not eating through the night. This is why breakfast is an essential meal for everyone, but especially for those in cancer treatment. It helps jump-start your morning and metabolism, and gives you a chance to load up on high-calorie, high-protein breakfast foods, such as a cheese omelet with a buttered bagel and a glass of 100-percent fruit juice, or a bowl of oatmeal made with milk (or commercial liquid supplement, such as Ensure or Boost), some honey or syrup, and a few teaspoons of butter. Eggs, yogurt, cheese, milk, wheat germ, and cottage cheese are some great protein additions to your breakfast.

- Eat by the clock and eat often. Look at a clock or your watch to help remind you that it's time to eat. Using a clock helps you rely on a schedule instead of your appetite. Focus on eating frequently and consistently and not on the quantity of what you are eating. Aim to eat or drink something every two to three hours. If your appetite becomes really compromised, and every bite of food seems to be a challenge, eat or drink something small that is packed with calories at least every hour. Even just a few small bites of something, such as a handful of nuts or a few crackers with cheese, or a few sips of high-calorie beverage, such as a milkshake or smoothie, adds up calories by the end of the day. Losing weight causes your stomach to become full more quickly than usual, which means it takes less food to make you feel full.

- Eat solid food first to avoid filling up on liquids, and drink most of your fluids between meals. If your parents told you not to drink with meals it's because liquids can fill up your stomach, leaving less room for the solid foods. Small sips with meals are okay, but avoid overdoing it. Also, avoid eating soup as a whole meal unless you are on an all liquid diet and instructed to do so, or it is a calorie-dense, thick, hearty, or creamy soup.

- Try high-calorie, high-protein drinks, such as commercial liquid supplements (Boost Plus, Ensure Plus, or Carnation Instant Breakfast VHC), nutritional bars, puddings, and homemade milkshakes (see Chapter 5). Use nutritional supplements between meals instead of substituting them for meals.

- Try eating all of your food on salad plates instead of dinner plates because the size of the plate is really the amount of food you should be eating at your "mini meals," and it's also more appealing to look at a smaller plate of food when your appetite is not great. Many patients have expressed to me that looking at a big plate filled with food can feel overwhelming and discouraging. If someone is helping you with food preparation, ask them to serve your food on smaller plates.

- Eat whatever foods you enjoy at any time of the day. For example, you can eat breakfast foods such as pancakes, waffles, French toast, or omelets for lunch or dinner, or eat dinner foods such as a hamburger in the morning if you're feeling up to it. Eat whatever you are in the mood to eat when you feel hungry. If you are feeling sick and nauseated, avoid your favorite foods so that you do not cause a food aversion.

- Ask your doctor for clearance to start some physical activity, such as light to moderate exercise, which can help promote appetite and maintain your muscle strength. Even just taking a short walk before meals can help increase your appetite. Start slow—add 10 minutes of activity per day and aim for at least 30 minutes of activity most days of the week. If you prefer to break up the 30 minutes, you can engage in three 10-minute bouts of light to moderate exercise. Moderate exercise not only helps prevent fatigue, but also helps promote bowel regularity.

- Many of my clients who want to lose weight tell me how they eat more food in social situations surrounded by friends and family. You may have noticed this happen with yourself in the past. The reason for this is because you are usually thinking less about what you're eating when you're distracted and engaged in a conversation; therefore, causing you to eat more without realizing it. For someone trying to gain weight, this can work in your favor. Creating a relaxed atmosphere with others will hopefully make you feel more at ease and less tense about food. If eating has become a challenge for you, eating among close friends and family may help take the burden of eating off of you for a little while. When you feel up to it, ask your friends and family to join you at meals, which can make eating a more positive and enjoyable experience. Also, try to combine different colored food, textures, and tastes on your plate to add even more appeal.

- Ever notice that when you bake or you smell someone else baking you suddenly become hungry? Pleasant aromas such as the smell of baking bread, cookies, or cake may help boost your appetite.

- Reach out to your friends and family for help with cooking and food shopping. Make shopping lists of the foods you enjoy eating right now and give it to them.

Weight loss

In simple terms, weight loss occurs when your body is using more calories than you are taking in. This means you are not taking in enough calories to keep up with your body's demands. You should be closely monitoring your weight on a scale during treatment to know if you are losing or gaining. Whether you choose to use a scale at home or at your treatment center, weigh yourself weekly to know if your weight is changing. It's important to use the same scale for continuity. If possible, weigh yourself at the same time every day and try to wear the same type of clothing and shoes (or remove your shoes every time). If you weigh yourself with clothes and shoes, you should subtract two to three pounds to account for the extra bulk. Keep track of your weekly weight in a small notebook. If you begin to lose weight, you should immediately start adjusting your diet to include foods higher in calories and protein. To reiterate what was discussed previously in this book, your body needs more calories and protein than usual during cancer treatment to help you maintain your weight, keep up your strength and energy, better tolerate the side effects of treatment, rebuild cells and tissue, and recover and heal as quickly as possible.

You may have even noticed that you've lost weight, even though you've been eating the same amount of food as usual. Having cancer, along with receiving treatment, changes your metabolism and increases your daily caloric needs, which means you need to eat more calories than usual each day to maintain your weight. Even if you changed nothing in your diet, and even before the start of treatment, you may experience weight loss due to an increased metabolic rate. For this reason, a person with cancer has a higher risk for unintentional weight loss and may need to adopt a high-calorie, high-protein diet even before treatment starts to help gain back some weight. Weight loss is also common during treatment because of the symptoms related to treatment, such as mouth sores, taste changes, poor appetite, nausea, difficulty swallowing, or shortness of breath, which make it challenging to eat enough calories.

The rule of thumb to gain or lose one pound of weight per week is to add or subtract approximately 500 calories per day. This means that if your goal is to gain one pound per week, you should add approximately 500 calories per day to what you are eating right now. This same concept applies to those who want to lose weight; it takes an average deficit of 500 calories per day to lose weight, so this can include eating less calories and exercising more to burn calories—for example, eat 300 calories less per day and exercise to burn off 200 calories. Most people have no idea how many calories they consume on a daily basis, so to make it easier for everyone, I tell my patients this: You don't need to know how many calories you are taking in. If you are losing weight, however many calories you are currently consuming on a daily basis is simply *not* enough to meet your caloric needs and is causing weight loss. Take whatever you are eating now and add in about 500 calories per day (spread throughout the day).

Ways to add calories to your diet

- Consume food and drinks that are not skimmed or reduced in fat, such as whole milk instead of skim milk and regular mayonnaise instead of reduced fat mayonnaise. Avoid drinks and food labeled as "low fat," "nonfat," or "diet." This may sound contradictory to the way you have been eating in the past, but remember that when you are losing weight, every single calorie counts! The extra 60 calories in a cup of whole milk versus a cup of skim milk and the extra 75 calories per tablespoon of real mayonnaise versus low-fat mayonnaise add up by the end of the day to help meet your total caloric needs.

- Snack attack! Choose calorie-dense snacks that contain many calories in a small amount. Some ideas are snacking on dried fruits, granola, and nuts and adding them to hot cereals, oatmeal, ice cream, yogurt, or salads. Grabbing small amounts of high-calorie foods can really help pack in the calories without taking up volume in your stomach. Just 1 ounce of almonds is 165 calories, one small box of raisins (1.5 ounces) is 130 calories, five dried apple rings is 80 calories, and one ounce of cheddar cheese is 110 calories. In the grocery store, compare food labels and check to see which foods have more calories per serving. For example, a 1/4 cup of regular granola cereal is about 150 calories, whereas one cup of Cheerios is 100 calories. This illustrates what it means to be a calorie-dense food. The granola contains far more calories per ounce, which allows you to eat more calories in a smaller amount. Cup for cup, you would get an extra 500 calories when you eat the granola versus the Cheerios. One cup of granola is about 600 calories. Mix granola into yogurt, with dried fruits and nuts, or sprinkle it on top of ice cream, custard, pudding, and fruit. You can also add granola into cookie, muffin, and bread recipes.

- Snack here, snack there, snack everywhere. Keep your favorite snack foods in your house and at work to eat when you are hungry, and don't forget to bring snacks to your appointments and when you travel. Some good snack ideas are cheese, crackers, yogurt, cereal and milk, trail mix, dried fruits, nuts, peanut butter, hard-boiled eggs, canned fruit, a bowl of hearty soup, granola bars, pudding, ice cream, frozen yogurt, liquid supplements, muffins, and power bars (PowerBar, Clif Bars, Balance Bars, Luna Bars, Odwalla Bars, NuGo Bars, or any others you enjoy). You can try your own homemade trail mix by combining your favorite nuts, seeds (pumpkin or sunflower), raisins or dried cranberries, and some dark chocolate chips, or buy a ready-to-eat trail mix.

- If you do not own a blender you should buy one. A blender is very useful for making homemade milkshakes and smoothies, which can really pack in the calories and help you gain weight. I list suggestions for recipe and smoothie ideas in the following chapter. You will see how using a little creativity and the right ingredients can create energy-dense shakes. Some of my most creative patients who were on liquid diets due to head and neck cancer created shakes and smoothies that were 1,000 calories each.

- Liberally add butter, margarine, oils, and gravies to rice, pastas, soups, cooked vegetables, mashed and baked potatoes, sandwiches, toast, hot cereals, and oatmeal. This is one of the best ways to sneak calories into the foods you are already eating. I love teaching my patients about this trick of sneaking calories into their diet because it gives people comfort to learn that they don't need to make drastic changes to their diets to gain weight. They just need to modify the foods they already enjoy eating. For example, instead of eating a plain baked potato, eat a baked potato topped with plenty of butter or margarine, sour cream, or cheddar cheese. Instead of eating a bowl of plain, cooked oatmeal, prepare the oatmeal with some butter or margarine; sugar, honey, or syrup; and stir in some milk, cream, or vanilla liquid supplement drink, such as Ensure or Boost.

- Spread cream cheese on vegetables, dip vegetables into a sour-cream based dip, or melt butter over vegetables.

- Drink high-calorie beverages such as hot chocolate, fruit juices, fruit nectars, milk, soy, or rice milk, sweetened iced tea, lemonade, Gatorade, Vitamin Water, Snapple, shakes, and smoothies. You can buy commercial smoothies when you're out and about, such as Odwalla and Naked smoothie drinks. Adequate hydration can be maintained by drinking 8 to 10 cups of fluids per day.

- Avoid filling up on low-calorie drinks such as water, coffee, tea, and diet drinks. These take up valuable space in your stomach and provide minimal calories. If you enjoy drinking coffee and tea, add whole milk or cream with honey or sugar for additional calories. Spread jelly, peanut butter, honey, butter, or cream cheese onto bread, toast, or crackers.

- Snack on tortilla chips dipped in guacamole or just cut up some avocado and chomp on a few slices for a snack. You can also add avocado to your sandwiches and salads for extra calories and healthy fat! Avocados contain the healthy mono- and polyunsaturated fats, such as omega-3 fatty acids, as well as dietary fiber, vitamins C and K, lutein (a carotenoid), and folate. One medium avocado is about 320 calories, making this another nutrient-dense food choice.

- Use high-calorie, regular dressings on salads, baked potatoes, or on chilled cooked vegetables such as green beans or asparagus. Pass on the reduced-fat and low-fat varieties. Just two tablespoons of most regular dressings is about 120–140 calories!

- Add sour cream, half-and-half, or heavy cream to mashed potatoes, cake and cookie recipes, sauces, gravies, soups, casseroles, cooked meat, stews, macaroni and cheese, and fish. Use sour cream as a dip for vegetables or fruit or as a topping for cakes, fruit, gelatin, breads, and muffins.

- Now is the time to indulge in whipped cream. Enjoy adding it to your foods and ordering it topped onto your favorite desserts, lattes, and hot chocolate. You can add whipped cream to desserts, ice cream, pancakes, waffles, fruit, and pudding.

- Prepare vegetables or pasta with cream sauces. Look for foods labeled as "creamed" when grocery shopping or ordering food from a restaurant, and choose creamy dishes at restaurants. Some good ideas are fettuccine alfredo, penne ala vodka, creamed vegetables, and creamed soups.

- Use mayonnaise in salads, on sandwiches, and in vegetable dips. One tablespoon of regular mayonnaise is 90 calories. Use it to prepare mayonnaise-based salads, such as egg salad, tuna salad, chicken salad, potato salad, and macaroni salad. Many people think the word "salad" implies that it is healthy and low-calorie. Many of my clients trying to lose weight tell me how they consider a tuna salad sandwich a good choice for their diet. I have to break the news that ordering a regular tuna salad sandwich (not reduced fat) can cost about 600–700 calories. For someone looking to gain weight, this is great news! Eating one half of a tuna salad, egg salad, or chicken salad sandwich would be a great idea for one of your mini-meals.

Quick Guide to High-Calorie Foods

Food	Portion	Calories
Half and half	1 tablespoon 1 cup	20 calories 320 calories
Sour cream	1 tablespoon	30 calories
Heavy cream	1 tablespoon	50 calories
Margarine or butter	1 tablespoon	100 calories
Mayonnaise	1 tablespoon	90 calories
Honey	1 tablespoon	65 calories
Syrups	2 tablespoons	80 calories
Dried fruits (raisins, prunes, dates, apricots, apple)	2/3 cup of raisins 1 cup of other dried fruit	300 calories varies from 200–400 calories
Granola	1/4 cup (1 ounce)	130 calories
Wheat germ	1/4 cup (1 ounce)	110 calories
Avocado	1/2 avocado	160 calories
Coconut (shredded)	13 tablespoons	115 calories

Ways to add protein to your diet

- Eat protein-rich foods such as chicken, beef, fish, eggs, cottage cheese, cheese, milk, hummus, beans, tofu, yogurt, Greek yogurt, nut butters (peanut butter, cashew butter), nuts, and wheat germ.
- Be cheesy. Snack on slices or cubes of cheese or on top of crackers or fruit. Add different cheeses, such as ricotta cheese, cottage cheese, parmesan cheese, and grated cheese, to omelets, soups, pastas, quiches,

baked and mashed potatoes, vegetables, and casseroles. Eat foods that contain cheese, such as manicotti,
lasagna, macaroni and cheese, quiches, and baked
ziti, and melt cheese onto hamburgers and breaded
chicken. One ounce (about the size of four dice) of
cheese is about 105 calories and 7 grams of protein.

- Drink "double strength milk" (see Chapter 5) or any
milk you prefer, and use it as a substitute in recipes
that call for milk or water, such as instant puddings,
hot chocolate, omelets, pancake and cake mixes,
cream soups, casseroles, and mashed potatoes.

- Add milk powder to cream soups, mashed potatoes,
milkshakes, casseroles, soufflés, and quiches. I refer
to powdered milk as the "cheaper protein supplement." The powder consists of milk protein, which is
an excellent protein source and can help supplement
your daily protein goals. You can find non-fat dry
milk powder packets in your supermarket.

- Add peanut butter or other nut butters, such as cashew butter, to fruits and vegetables (apples, bananas,
and celery), desserts, sandwiches, crackers, and milkshakes, or simply scoop it right out of the jar with a
spoon and eat it plain. Just two tablespoons is 190 calories, 8 grams of protein, and contains heart-healthy
fats. Snacking on nuts is another great calorie-filled
snack. A handful of nuts contains about 200 calories
and 8 grams of protein too!

- Add cooked chicken or meat to soups, casseroles,
omelets, salads, and quiches. For high-protein vegetarian options, add beans, chickpeas, lentils, and tofu
to salads, soups, casseroles, and vegetable dishes. Try
hummus with pita bread or crackers. You can also
sprinkle wheat germ into yogurt, casseroles, farina,
cereal, and oatmeal.

- Eggs are a great source of protein as they provide all of the essential amino acids for humans, and contain several vitamins and minerals, such as vitamins A, D, and E, B12, and folate. One egg contains about 80 calories and 7 grams of protein. Eat desserts prepared with eggs, such as custards, cheesecake, and angel food cake. Keep hard-boiled eggs in the refrigerator and chop them up and add to salads, casseroles, and soups. Use them to make egg salad. As discussed previously, *never* eat raw eggs because of the risk of salmonella poisoning, which is one of the food-borne illnesses.

- Feel free to add pasteurized liquid egg products, such as Egg Beaters, to soups, stews, and mashed potatoes. Add pasteurized powdered egg whites to milk, milkshakes, soups, and mashed potatoes.

- You can also try protein supplements, which are complete protein sources, such as the unflavored powder, Beneprotein (go to *www.nestlenutritionstore.com* or call 1-888-240-2713) or Unjury flavored and unflavored powder (go to *www.unjury.com/store/protein* or call 1-800-517-5111).

Quick Guide to Protein Foods

Food	Portion	Calories	Protein
Eggs	1 medium	80 calories	7 grams
Egg substitutes (pasteurized)	1/4 cup	55 calories	8 grams
Cheese	1 ounce	100 calories	7–8 grams
Parmesan cheese, grated	1/4 cup	110 calories	10 grams

Milk	8 ounces	Whole: 150 calories Skim: 90 calories	8 grams
Non-fat milk powder	1/4 cup	110 calories	11 grams
4% creamed cottage cheese	1 cup	220 calories	30 grams
Ice cream	1 cup	Low-fat: 150 calories Premium, rich, regular: 270	5 grams
Yogurt (vanilla or plain whole milk)	8 ounce	150 calories	7 grams
Yogurt (fruit flavored, low-fat)	8 ounce	250 calories	11 grams
Greek yogurt	6 ounces	110–240 calories (depends on brand)	11–15 grams (depends on brand)
Beef, pork, poultry, fish	1 ounce cooked	75 calories	7 grams
Peanut butter or nut spreads	2 tablespoons	190 calories	9 grams
Nuts (dry roasted)	1 ounce	160–180 calories	7 grams
Tofu	1/2 cup	95 calories	10 grams

Legumes, beans (cooked)	1/2 cup	100 calories	7 gram
Tuna (canned)	3 ounces	Oil packed: 170 calories Water packed: 110 calories	25 grams
Soy milk, plain	1 cup	100 calories	7 grams
Soybeans (edamame)	1/2 cup cooked	150 calories	14 grams
Tempeh	1/2 cup	165 calories	16 grams
Frozen yogurt, vanilla	1 cup	250	7

? ## Should I try nutritional supplements, such as Ensure or Boost?

If you are losing weight, you can supplement your diet with commercial liquid supplements that are ready-to-use and easy to transport with you to appointments, or you can add them to homemade milkshakes (see Chapter 5). These supplements may also be very helpful for those who can only tolerate mostly pureed and liquid food due to mouth soreness. Liquid supplements can be used alone or in any shake or smoothie recipe, and often come in a variety of flavors. Many of the supplements are lactose-free, are fortified with vitamins and minerals, and are available in higher-calorie varieties ("plus" varieties), such Ensure Plus or Boost Plus. Choose plus versions if weight loss is significant and you have early fullness. Some examples of liquid supplements on the market include: Nutren (Nestlè), Ensure (Abbott), Boost (Nestlè), Carnation Instant Breakfast Drink (Nestlè), Glucerna

(Abbott), Nepro (Abbott), Boost Glucose Control (Nestlè), Osmolite (Abbott), and Isosource (Nestlè). There are also fruity drink supplements that are lactose-free, fat-free, and clear liquid, such as Enlive (Abbott) and Resource Breeze (Nestlè), for those who prefer fruit flavored drinks or those who better tolerate clear liquids. Milk-based powdered supplements are also available and can also be mixed into shakes, milk, or water, such as Carnation Instant Breakfast and Scandishake packets, and come in different flavors and sugar-free varieties. As a caveat, I caution against using any of these commercial supplements as *substitutes* for meals. As the word "*supplement*" implies, these should be used in addition to the foods you are eating. Unless you are instructed to be on a complete liquid diet and drink these supplements as meals, I suggest you use them between meals and after eating solid foods. Talk to the dietitian at your treatment center to discuss if supplements are right for you and which ones would be most beneficial. Your cancer center or dietitian may have free samples for you try before purchasing.

If you would like to purchase any of the ready-to-use supplements, you can check your local supermarket or drug store to see if they carry the brand you are interested in buying. If they don't carry the product you want to buy, you can contact the company or order online:

- **Abbott Nutrition:** *www.abbottnutrition.com* 1-800-258-7677

- **Nestle Nutrition:** *www.nestlenutritionstore.com* 1-888-281-6400

- **Axcan Pharma:** *www.axcan.com/us_scandishake.php* 1-800-472-2634

You can also buy ready-to-drink shakes and smoothies when you're on the go and you need a high-calorie drink, but don't have a blender to make your own shakes and smoothies. For those who tolerate mostly liquids, these drinks can come in handy if you don't have supplements with you and you are away from home. Some examples are: Tropicana Smoothie, Hershey's Cream Shakes, Nesquik drink, Odwalla, Naked, and Stoneyfield smoothies, and any restaurant or ice cream store's shakes, sundaes, or smoothies. You can also get a milkshake at McDonald's, Dairy Queen, Dunkin' Donuts, or a frappuccino (made with whole milk) at Starbuck's. Treat yourself to these now, because when you finish treatment and maintain a healthy weight, you should avoid drinking high- calorie milkshakes.

Sore mouth or throat

Some cancer treatments can sometimes cause your mouth or throat to become very sore and make it hard to eat, chew, and swallow. This is referred to as *mucositis*. You should speak with your doctor or nurse about medications available to help with sore mouth. In terms of what you can eat that won't irritate your mouth or throat, the suggestions below can help you better enjoy eating and assist your mouth and throat with healing. To help prevent mucositis and heal mouth sores, it is crucial to maintain good oral hygiene and practice good oral care. One key tip to keep your mouth clean is to rinse your mouth often and after meals with a homemade rinse (1 quart water, 3/4 teaspoon salt, and 1 teaspoon baking soda). You should rinse and spit after each meal and, if needed, before meals. Swishing and spitting cleans germs and food out of your mouth, which in turn helps the healing process and prevents mouth infections.

Ways to eat and drink to manage sore or irritated mouth or throat

- Choose soft, well-moistened, and bland foods that are easier to chew or swallow and cause less irritation. If you notice you are starting to lose a little weight, begin incorporating higher-calorie, soft foods. Some high-calorie soft food ideas include: cream soups, stews, pasta with cream sauces, melted cheese, mashed potatoes with gravy, scrambled eggs, hot cooked cereal (farina, Cream of Wheat), grits, or oatmeal made with whole milk or a vanilla liquid supplement, macaroni and cheese, casseroles, yogurt, pudding, custard, ice cream, guacamole, bread stuffing, shakes and smoothies, syrup, gravies, tenderly cooked chicken, beef, or fish, and mayonnaise-based salads such as egg salad, tuna salad, chicken salad, and macaroni salad.

- Cut your food into smaller, bite-size pieces to make it easier to chew and swallow.

- Serve foods cold, at room temperature, or lukewarm. Hot foods may irritate the mouth or throat.

- Try chilled and cold foods and beverages, which can be soothing. You can freeze fruits to eat or suck, such as grapes, banana pieces, melon and cantaloupe balls, or peach slices. Try sucking on popsicles, fruit ices, ice chips, or other cold foods. Other soothing cold foods are milkshakes, smoothies, yogurt, gelatin, custard, and cottage cheese.

- You may feel more comfortable eating soft, pureed, or liquid foods that have a smoother consistency and are easier to eat and swallow. This may be especially helpful for fruits, vegetables, chunky soups, and meats. You can puree or liquefy solid foods using a blender, food processor, or immersion hand blender, or you can buy baby food. Solid foods like cooked meat, chicken, fish, pasta, potatoes, soups, rice, fruits, vegetables, and even mixed dishes, such as stews and casseroles, can be blended with liquids—whole milk, cream, baby food, gravies, cream sauces, vegetable juices, fruit juices, or broth. After blending, strain if necessary.

- Using a straw to drink all liquids and pureed foods may help increase your food intake by allowing food to bypass the sores in your mouth. Another trick that may help is to tilt your head back to help foods and liquids flow towards your throat, helping you swallow more easily.

- Eat "wet" foods that are moistened well. You can moisten foods with any liquids, including soups, sauces, broth, milk, juice, yogurt, jelly, gravy, and olive or canola oil. You can soften any food by dipping or soaking it in any warm or cold liquid you enjoy. Try cookies or cakes dipped in milk or coffee, a roll soaked in your favorite soup, or pancakes or waffles moistened with maple syrup.

- Drink at least 8 to 10 cups (1 cup = 8 ounces) of caffeine-free beverages each day. Carry a water bottle with you and sip on it throughout the day.

- Make smoothies with fruits such as melons, bananas, peaches, pears, and nectarines (peel the skin before blending) and mix with frozen yogurt, ice cream, milk, yogurt, milk, or tofu for extra protein. Avoid fruits that contain small seeds, which can irritate the mouth, such as strawberries, blueberries, or blackberries. You can also buy commercial smoothies, such as Stonyfield yogurt smoothies.

- If you suffer from gastric reflux and heartburn, stop eating two to three hours before bedtime and sleep with your head elevated. You should raise the head of your bed about 6–9 inches by putting a foam wedge under the top part of the mattress or placing blocks of wood under the legs of the head of your bed. Avoid chocolate, alcohol, smoking, spearmint and peppermint, caffeinated beverages (tea, coffee, and cola), citrus fruits (orange, lemon, lime, and grapefruit), spicy foods, tomato-based foods, raw garlic and onions, and high-fat and fried foods. Wearing loose-fitting clothes may also be helpful.

- Talk to your doctor about medications that can soothe and numb your mouth or throat, such as "magic mouthwash," Gelcair, UlcerEase, or Orabase. "Magic mouthwash" preparations must be prescribed by your physician, are used to swish and spit at least four to six times per day, and help clean and temporarily provide numbing relief to your mouth.

? What should I avoid eating if I have a sore mouth?

- Avoid very tart, acidic, or salty foods and beverages that can cause irritation. Some of these food include:
  - citrus fruits (oranges, grapefruit, limes, pineapple, lemons).
  - fruits with small seeds (berries).
  - pickled and vinegary foods (relishes and pickles).
  - tomato-based foods, such as salsa, ketchup, marinara sauce, chili, and pizza.
  - broths (canned and dry packets).
- Avoid irritating spices, seasonings, and condiments, such as pepper and pepper sauces, chili powder, cloves, curry, mustard, hot sauces, barbeque sauce, Worcestershire sauce, nutmeg, and horseradish.
- Avoid rough, dry foods with sharp edges which can scratch your mouth or throat. Some examples are dry toast, crackers, chips, pretzels, granola, tough meats, and raw fruits and vegetables.

- Avoid commercial mouthwashes, acidic beverages, and tobacco (cigarettes, pipes, and chewing tobacco). They can irritate and dry your mouth.
- Avoid alcoholic beverages, such as beer, wine, and mixed drinks.

Maintaining oral care

Keeping your mouth healthy and clean plays an important role in keeping you healthy during cancer treatment and recovery, and helps prevent mouth infections, mouth sores, and cavities. Chemotherapy and radiation therapy can cause a sore mouth or throat, making you more susceptible to serious mouth infections and causing pain when eating. Therefore, routine oral care is not something that you should overlook. You may be instructed to visit your dentist before, during, or after your cancer treatment.

Suggestions for good oral care

- Gently floss your teeth at least twice a day. Do not floss if your platelet count is low or if it causes bleeding or pain. Your doctor or nurse will tell you if your platelet count is low.
- Gently brush your teeth with a soft or extra-soft toothbrush within 30 minutes after eating a meal or snack, as well as before bedtime (a minimum of four times per day). Be sure to brush your teeth and rinse your mouth after eating or drinking foods or beverages with high sugar content, such as milkshakes or ice cream.
- Use toothpaste that contains fluoride and apply fluoride gel on your teeth before bedtime.
- Rinse your mouth *before and after* eating with a homemade mouth rinse that can be made my mixing together 1 quart warm or cold water, 3/4 teaspoon salt, and 1 teaspoon baking soda until the baking soda

and salt dissolve. Rinse with this solution at least four to six times per day and follow the solution with a plain water rinse. It is especially important to rinse after eating meals and anything sugary to prevent infections and sores. If your mouth is sore, avoid mouth rinses that contain alcohol. If your mouth is very sore, rinse your mouth with the homemade solution every one to two hours, as well as with "magic mouthwash" that your doctor can prescribe.

- Soak your toothbrush in warm water for a minute before using to help soften the bristles. You can also use a foam swab (Toothette) to clean teeth; however, if you have severe mucositis, a toothbrush or Toothette may be too harsh to use and you should instead use one of the recommended rinses to cleanse your mouth.

- If you have dentures, only wear them when you are eating. Be sure to brush them and keep them clean. Clean them in effervescent denture cleansers and rinse well before wearing.

- Keep your lips moisturized by using lip balm, petroleum jelly, or cocoa butter. Do not share these items with others.

- Drink plenty of fluids throughout the day to keep your mouth moisturized and wet. If your mouth is dry, chew sugarless gum or suck on sugarless hard candy. You can also try water-based mouth moisturizers. More tips for dry mouth are listed in the next section.

Dry mouth and thick saliva

Your mouth may become dry from radiation therapy, chemotherapy, medications, head and neck surgery, fever, dehydration, or infections. The medical term for dry mouth is *xerostomia*. Dry mouth occurs as a result of your salivary glands producing less saliva. Depending on your treatment, you may also experience thick saliva that may feel sticky or stringy in your mouth and throat. If you experience extreme mouth dryness, you should be aware that this can cause problems with chewing, swallowing, tasting, eating, talking, and sleeping. You are also at higher risk for cavities or mouth infections because saliva helps keep your mouth clean and protects your teeth from decay, so keep your mouth clean by following the previous oral care recommendations. You should visit your dentist before, during, and after treatment. It is very important for you to alert your medical team if symptoms arise so you can receive the best management for dry mouth. If it is hard for you to swallow or talk, you may need to meet with a speech pathologist to help improve these issues.

Similar to the suggestion for mouth soreness, you will be more comfortable eating moist, soft foods to help keep your mouth as moist and soothed as possible. To avoid worsening mouth dryness, avoid smoking, chewing tobacco, or drinking alcoholic beverages. A key tip for dry mouth and thick saliva management is to drink up! Drinking plenty of fluids throughout the day helps loosen thick secretions. You may need to drink more fluids than you were accustomed to drinking before. Caffeine-free drinks are the best option because caffeinated drinks such as coffee, teas, cola can worsen dry mouth. Some people find it soothing to sip on warm, caffeine-free tea. If you are also losing weight, drinks should contain calories, but be sure to swish and spit with water or the mouth rinse (as described previously) right after you finish your drink. You don't want to let any sugary drinks sit in your mouth for too long.

Ways to eat and drink to manage dry mouth and thick saliva

- Eat mainly soft, pureed, and bland foods that are room temperature. See page 83 for more suggestions on softening your foods.

- To help drink the recommended 8 to 12 cups of caffeine-free liquids a day, try carrying a water bottle filled with your favorite drink wherever you go and sip on it frequently.

- To help stimulate your saliva, chew sugarless gum or suck on sugar-free citrus candy, such as sugar-free lemon drops. Drinks and candies that contain citrus may also help promote saliva.

- To help stimulate saliva, try very sour or sweet foods and citrus drinks, such as lemon juice, lemonade, or cranberry juice. Try sucking on a cherry or olive pit or the rind of a lemon or lime. However, if you have mouth sores, avoid sour and acidic food and drinks.

- Cut your food into small pieces, eat slowly, and chew thoroughly.

- Try fresh or canned fruits that contain plenty of water in them, such as watermelon, peaches, nectarines, grape, and oranges.

- Avoid salty or spicy foods that can make your thirsty and irritate your mouth.

- Eat cold foods and beverages that can help soothe and moisten your mouth, such as milkshakes, ice cream, sorbet, frozen yogurt, smoothies, yogurt, gelatin, cottage cheese, and pureed fruits and vegetables. Try sucking on frozen fruit pops, fruit ices, and ice chips. You can also freeze fruits such as grapes, cantaloupe cubes, sliced peaches, sliced watermelon, banana slices, and orange slices.

- Sip on 100-percent papaya or pineapple juice alone or with club soda. The natural ingredients in these fruits can help thin out your saliva.

- Avoid dry meats without sauces; dry breads; crumbly foods such as crackers, chips, and pretzels; cereals not moistened in liquids; and raw vegetables.

- Some people find that milk contributes to mucous, so avoid milk if it causing too much mucous.

- Avoid small particle foods that can cause choking, such as rice and peas.

? What are some of the products available to treat dry mouth and diminished saliva production?

There are products available that you can buy at many drugstores, but you may need to ask the pharmacist to get it for you behind the counter. You should also discuss with your doctor or nurse the medical management of dry mouth and thick saliva because they may suggest that you take a prescription medication, such as Salagen (Pilocarpine) or Evoxac (Cevimiline) that stimulates the production of saliva. Ask your pharmacist about products made for dry mouth, such as saliva substitutes and mouth moisturizers. Some examples are Oral Balance, Xero-lube, Mouth Kote, Salivart, Moi-Stir, Optimoist, or Glandosane.

If you would like to buy a non-prescription mouthwash, avoid choosing one that contains alcohol, such as Listerine and Scope, and instead try an alcohol-free mouthwash, such as Biotene. Remember, you can always make your own mild homemade mouth rinse with 1 teaspoon baking soda and 3/4 teaspoon salt dissolved into 1 quart of water. Biotene also makes other great products that are appropriate for dry and sore mouth during treatment, such as antibacterial toothpaste and antibacterial gum.

Taste and smell changes

The taste and smell of food is often closely related to your appetite. If you are experiencing a loss of taste, this can take away the pleasure of eating, causing your appetite to decline. The four basic taste sensations are sweet, sour, bitter, and salty. Using the taste buds on your tongue, you can sense the taste of foods.

Smelling the aroma of foods further enhances your sensation of taste. Taste and smell work hand-in-hand to provide you the pleasure of eating. Temporary taste, smell, and appetite changes are common results of some cancer treatments, such as chemotherapy and radiation therapy. Chemotherapy affects all rapidly dividing cells in your body, including your taste buds, which is why it can decrease the activity of your taste buds. Chemotherapy and radiation to the head or neck area can affect your salivary glands, which causes decreased saliva production and a dry mouth, thereby decreasing your sensation of taste.

You should be aware that your taste and smell senses can change from day to day, so try to be creative and open-minded, and experiment with new foods or cuisines, marinades, and spices. Foods may taste bland, chalky, metallic, too sweet, bitter, or have little taste. Please note, if you cannot eat for more than a day because of taste changes, call your doctor or nurse. The loss of taste and smell is typically temporary and usually picks up again within several months following the end of your treatment. It may take longer than that for some people, so do not be alarmed if this side effect lasts for months after treatment ends.

Ways to eat and drink to manage taste and smell changes

- Avoid foods with strong odors. Choose low odor and non-bitter foods, such as French toast, pancakes, oatmeal, cream of wheat, cereal, shakes, smoothies, bread, pasta, fruit nectars, yogurt, frozen fruit, and ice pops. If red meat is unappealing, choose alternative sources of protein such as chicken, turkey, mild fish, eggs, beans, tofu, peanut butter, nuts, seeds, cottage cheese, and yogurt.
- If meat or chicken tastes funny to you, try marinating and cooking meats in sweet juices, fruits, salad dressings (Italian dressing), wine, mustard, or barbeque,

soy, or teriyaki sauce. Some ideas are sweet-and-sour chicken with pineapple, sweet-and-sour meatballs, or chicken with a teriyaki sauce or a cranberry glaze. You can also add sauces and condiments to other foods.

- Experiment with different herbs and spices to enhance the flavor and smell of foods. You can increase the amount of spices in recipes if it seems to be helping your taste buds. Depending on what appeals to you, try adding basil, oregano, rosemary, tarragon, thyme, mustard, ketchup, vanilla, almond flavoring, and mint. You can also try experimenting with strong flavors if the smell doesn't bother you, such as onion, garlic, and feta and parmesan cheeses. If your mouth is irritated, avoid ground chili, curry, pepper, and large amounts of salt.

- Try seasoning your foods with tart and sour flavors, such as lemon, lime, lemon juice, citrus fruits, cranberries, cranberry juice, vinegar, or pickled foods (avoid if you mouth or throat is sore). These flavors can mask bitter or metallic tastes.

- Suck on sugar-free candies, such as lemon drops, mints, or other hard sugar-free candy, and chew sugarless mint gum.

- Cold or room temperature foods may be easier to eat than warm foods because they tend to have less odors.

- If cooking food bothers you, ask friends or family to bring you prepared food, or avoid the kitchen when someone else is cooking. You can also prepare meals and snacks that do not need to be cooked and require less time in the kitchen, such as cold sandwiches, crackers and cheese, yogurt, fruit, granola, or cold cereal and milk.

- If your food tastes too salty, bitter, or sour, try adding a little bit of sugar or something sweet. If something tastes very sweet, try adding lemon juice or salt.

- If you have a metallic taste in your mouth, try using plastic utensils instead of metal; choose fresh or frozen foods instead of canned foods; and use glass or ceramic cookware.

- Experiment with different homemade shake recipes (see Chapter 5). Try frozen fruits, such as whole grapes and mandarin orange slices, or chopped cantaloupe or watermelon.

- Rinse your mouth before eating with one of the cleansing solutions discussed on page 89 to clean your taste buds before eating. You can also try rinsing with cool black or green tea.

- Drink from a straw or use a cup with a lid. Try this when drinking liquid supplements, such as Ensure or Boost Plus, that can sometimes smell unpleasant to people.

- Avoid your favorite foods if you are not feeling well as this can cause an acquired food aversion.

- Supplemental zinc may help with taste sensations. Low levels of zinc are associated with decreased taste sensation. Discuss with your doctor or dietitian if you should supplement with zinc.

Nausea and vomiting

Nausea and vomiting can be a side effect of chemotherapy or radiation therapy, medications (opiods such as codeine or oxycodone), bowel obstruction, infection, peptic ulcers, intense pain, fatigue, or anxiety that can interfere with eating well and cause weight loss, dehydration, metabolic problems, and electrolyte imbalances if not properly managed. If you experience vomiting, immediately discuss this with your doctor or nurse because it is dangerous if not treated in a timely manner. Dehydration can occur quickly if you are vomiting. Medications used to treat nausea and/or vomiting are called *antiemetics,* and they can be used preventively, routinely for several days after chemotherapy, or as needed. If you are receiving radiation to your chest, abdomen, brain, or pelvis, nausea and vomiting may start within one to two hours after receiving treatment and may continue for a few hours. There are many highly effective drugs that prevent and control nausea; if one medication does not seem to help, ask your doctor if a different medication would work better. The occurrence and treatment for nausea and vomiting depends on the person, the type of treatment, and the underlying cause. It's important to try to control nausea and vomiting as soon as possible with medication because nausea can cause and worsen weight loss. Weight loss occurs because people have much less desire to eat when they are nauseated, and the diet suggestions for nausea include eating low-fat foods which are lower in calories.

Ways to eat and drink to manage nausea and vomiting

- Have someone else prepare your meals and bring them to you or order take-out foods from restaurants because the smell of cooking can lead to increased nausea. You can also prepare meals ahead of time, freeze them in single portions, and reheat them on the days you don't feel well. This is especially helpful on days after chemotherapy when you are most likely to experience nausea. Ask your doctor or nurse if your treatment is likely to cause nausea and how long it is likely to last. Sometimes nausea can be delayed for a few days after treatment.

- Eat a small, light meal before you come to chemotherapy or radiation therapy, unless your health care team directs you otherwise. Eat small, frequent snacks and meals high- carbohydrate, low-fat, low-fiber foods that are easy to digest and have minimal odors, such as crackers, pretzels, bagels, dry cereals, dry white bread or toast (unbuttered), soft breads, breadsticks, angel food cake, vanilla wafers, oatmeal, farina, baked or boiled potatoes (without butter), plain noodles, white rice, skinless chicken or turkey (white meat), mild soups, applesauce, canned unsweetened fruit, gelatin, ice pops, sherbet, frozen yogurt, and low-fat ice cream. The quicker that food passes from your stomach into your intestines, the less likely you are to experience nausea and vomiting. High-fat and high-fiber foods sit in your stomach for many hours and are slower to digest. Stay away from uncooked fruits and vegetables on days you feel nauseated. Convenient, single-serving foods, such as granola bars, yogurt, pudding, pretzels, crackers, breadsticks, canned fruit, gelatin, or applesauce, are easy options for when you're away from home.

- Try cold, room-temperature, or warm foods and see what makes you feel better. If cold foods give you comfort, you can suck on frozen fruit, such as watermelon, peaches, grapes, strawberries, and cherries, ice chips, frozen ices, ice pops, and sorbets or drink ice water and iced tea. If warm foods give you comfort, you can eat warm, bland foods such as soup or farina.

- Be careful of dehydration. Drink small sips of clear fluids throughout the day, such as fruit juice, sport drinks, slushies, water, cool broth, flat soda, hot tea and iced tea, all of which can help hydrate you. Anything that melts at room temperature is considered a fluid that can hydrate you (ice pops, ice chips). Drink most of your liquids between meals. If possible, try sipping liquids every few minutes. If you are losing weight, drink more of the fluids that contain calories like sport drinks, fruit juices, flat soda, and slushies.

- Avoid fried, greasy, rich, and very spicy foods, high-fiber whole-wheat products, and carbonated drinks. Greasy foods are harder to digest and stay in your stomach longer. Some foods to include fried eggs, french fries, heavy cream soups, creamed vegetables, pastries, doughnuts, cookies, potato chips, butter, salad dressing, peanut butter, nuts, milk, cheese, meats, bacon, sausage, and deli meat. Avoid spicy foods made with pepper, chili pepper, onion, or hot sauce. Spicy foods can aggravate your stomach, and carbonated drinks can cause gas and bloating. If you wish to have carbonated beverages, open them and let them stand for 10 minutes before drinking.

- Avoid eating odorous foods such as garlic, onions, peppers, horseradish, hard-boiled eggs, fish, broccoli, cabbage, cauliflower, and brussels sprouts. Try foods that have little odor, such as scrambled eggs, french toast, pancakes, oatmeal, cream of wheat, cold cereal, canned fruit, and shakes and smoothies (see Chapter 5).

- Watch out for gas-producing foods, such as beans, corn, peas, chives, cucumbers, leeks, peppers, radishes, sauerkraut, carbonated drinks, melons, apricots, prunes, raw apples, wheat bran, and artificial sweeteners and sugar alcohols (NutraSweet, Splenda, mannitol, xylitol, and sorbitol).

- Ginger may help prevent nausea. You can sip on ginger tea (see Chapter 5), suck on ginger candy, or add chopped, fresh ginger root or dried ginger to your foods. Enjoy foods with ginger such as ginger snaps, ginger ale, and crystallized ginger.

- Eat sitting up and do not recline for at least one to two hours after eating.

- Eat slowly and chew your food well.

- Try sucking on hard candies such as mints and lemon drops that can counteract a bad taste in your mouth. Mint teas may be soothing.

- Avoid strong perfumes, colognes, aftershaves, and scented body lotions. Try fragrance-free products for soaps and detergents, if needed. Ask friends and family to avoid wearing perfume or cologne if it bothers you.

- Keep your mouth clean by brushing your teeth and flossing.

- To remove bad tastes, rinse your mouth before eating with the homemade rinse listed on page 89.

- Try drinking from an insulated travel mug that has a lid that can block smells that cause nausea. You can put any liquids into the covered mug, including soups, broths, and liquid supplements such as Boost or Ensure. You can also drink the supplement through a straw in a lidded cup.

- If you vomit, rinse your mouth with water and brush your teeth to get the taste out of your mouth. Do not eat or drink anything for at least 30 minutes to let your stomach settle down. If the nausea has passed after 30 minutes, try a small sip or two of water, apple juice, cranberry juice, flat soda, broth, or flavored ices. Wait 15 minutes before trying a little more water or liquid. Continue taking small amounts with breaks and gradually increase the amount you drink each time. If your nausea subsides after two hours, try eating one or two crackers. Stick to eating very small amounts of food often (one or two bites of bland food or a clear liquid drink every hour).

- Do not take your medications on an empty stomach unless your doctor or pharmacist tells you to do so. You can have a piece of toast, some cereal, or a few crackers when you wake up.

- If you are feeling nauseated, cool yourself down by opening a window, turning on a fan, or going outside. You can put an ice pack or cold cloth on your neck and/or forehead.

Diarrhea

Cancer treatments can cause diarrhea, which is commonly defined as having two or more very loose or watery (liquidy) stools per day. Most often, diarrhea is caused by chemotherapy drugs, radiation therapy to the prostate, cervix, intestine, rectum or pancreas, and surgery on the stomach, intestine, or pancreas, all of which can lead to maldigestion and malabsorption of nutrients. Diarrhea means that food is moving too quickly through your digestive system, and you are not absorbing nutrients and water well. Uncontrolled diarrhea can be very dangerous if not treated with dietary changes, medications, or both, and can lead to severe stomach cramping, weakness, poor appetite, dehydration, weight loss, and electrolyte abnormalities. In addition to following the nutrition tips listed here, ask your doctor or nurse if you should be taking an anti-diarrheal medication and which one is right for you. Be sure to immediately call your doctor if your diarrhea persists for more than two days, your stools have an usual color or odor, there is blood in your stool, you have fever, your abdomen becomes swollen, or you lose more than 2 pounds in one to two days.

The first thing you can do if you have diarrhea is to make some dietary changes. The foods and drinks you consume can really help control diarrhea. You should immediately remove foods from your diet that may worsen diarrhea. Foods that can aggravate diarrhea include foods high in insoluble fiber, such as nuts, seeds, raw fruits and vegetables, dried fruits, whole grains (brown rice, whole-wheat bread, wheat bran), and legumes. Other foods that may contribute to diarrhea include high-fat, greasy, fried foods, such as french fries and doughnuts.

Ways to eat and drink to manage diarrhea

- The loss of fluids from diarrhea can cause dehydration, so drink plenty of fluids to replace lost fluids. Some signs of dehydration include: dry mouth, dry skin, dark yellow urine, feeling thirstier than usual, less frequent urination, and a weight loss of several pounds in one to two days. Drink at least 8 to 10 cups of liquids per day. Focus on drinking mild, clear liquids that are room temperature, but drink slowly and don't drink too much at once. Sip small amounts of liquids all day (at least 1/2 cup every hour), and try to drink most of your liquids between meals. Avoid fluids that contain caffeine, such as caffeinated coffee, tea, and colas, carbonated beverages, and alcohol. You can drink carbonated beverages that have been left open for at least 10 minutes before drinking.

- Choose water, plain broth, flat soda and seltzer, decaffeinated tea, sports drinks (Gatorade and Powerade), diluted juices, and fruit nectars such as apricot, peach, or pear (dilute with half water, half juice). Avoid apple, prune, and grape juices. Drink at least 1 cup of liquid after every loose bowel movement.

- For more severe diarrhea, replace water and electrolytes with coconut water, Pedialyte, CeraLyte, G2, and diluted sports drink (Gatorade and Powerade) with a 50/50 mix of water to sport drink.

- Eat small snacks all day long instead of large meals to allow your body time to digest foods.

- Eat foods plain, boiled, broiled, or steamed. Choose low-fat, bland foods, and foods that contain soluble fiber, including:
    - Oatmeal, oat bran, Cream of Rice, farina, Rice Krispies, cornflakes, cornbread.

- White rice, plain pasta, pastina, white bread, matzohs, white English muffins, rice cakes.

- Pretzels, crackers, saltines, graham crackers.

- Bananas, banana flakes, applesauce, peeled apples, well-cooked and peeled vegetables (beets, carrots, acorn or summer squash, turnips, green beans), and canned or cooked fruits without the skins.

- Mild soups (chicken soup with rice or noodles; no cream soups).

- Baked, boiled, steamed, or poached lean meats, such as skinless chicken or turkey (white meat) fish; smooth peanut butter (in small amounts); egg whites (gradually add egg yolks), Egg Beaters.

- Baked, mashed, or boiled potatoes (without skin or butter)

- Gelatin, ice pops, sherbet

- Non-fat or low-fat yogurt (contains active cultures called probiotics which help improve digestion).

- Sprinkle nutmeg on foods, which can slow down intestinal activity.

- With your doctor's permission, you can try to use commercial powders that contain psyllium fiber (a soluble fiber that helps absorb water and thicken your stool), such as Metamucil or Benefiber. These are over-the-counter products that don't require a prescription.

- Drink and eat salty foods to replace lost sodium, such as broths, soups, sport drinks, saltines, and pretzels, to help retain fluids in your body.

- Drink and eat high-potassium foods to replace lost potassium such as sports drinks; fruits juices and nectars (diluted); boiled, baked, or mashed potatoes (without the skin); and bananas.

- Include foods that contain *probiotics* which are good bacteria for your intestines found in fermented dairy products, such as yogurt, acidophilus milk, and kefir. Many yogurts on the market even have extra probiotics added.

- Talk to your doctor or dietitian about taking a standard daily multivitamin with minerals if you are following a diet with limited amounts of fruits, vegetables, and whole grains for a while.

? What foods should I avoid if I have diarrhea?

As stated previously, there are some foods that can worsen diarrhea (which makes food pass more quickly through your intestines). Here are some tips to help avoid this:

- Avoid greasy, fried, spicy, creamy, or very sweet foods. Limit margarine, butter, and oils during this time.

- Avoid dairy products if they seem to aggravate your diarrhea, such as milk, ice cream, and cheese, or try taking supplemental lactase (the enzyme that digests milk sugar) in the form of Lactaid or Dairy-Ease pills when you eat dairy. You can also try switching to lactose-free milk products, such as Lactaid and Dairy-Ease, or drinking soy or rice milk.

- Limit large quantities of sugar and foods containing artificial sweeteners and sugar alcohols (sorbitol, xylitol, and mannitol). Sugar alcohols are found in sugar-free foods, gums, candies, and mints. These can cause diarrhea, gas, and bloating.

- Avoid raw fruits and vegetables (especially "gassy" veggies such as broccoli, cauliflower, cabbage, beans, brussels sprouts, corn, peas, peppers, and onions) and dried fruits.

- Avoid nuts and seeds.

- Avoid extremely hot or cold foods.

- Avoid tobacco in all forms (cigarettes, pipe, and chewing tobacco) and alcohol.

Constipation

Constipation is a decrease in the normal frequency of your bowel movements, difficulty passing stools, or having hard stools. It can be a side effect of some chemotherapy, anti-nausea and pain medications, lack of physical activity, lack of eating, not getting enough fiber, and not drinking enough fluids. One of the best ways to ease constipation is to increase the amount of fiber and fluids at each meal. If changing your eating habits doesn't help, you may need to take bowel medications such as stool softeners, laxatives, or enemas to keep your bowel movements regular and soft. Before taking any over-the-counter products, check first with your doctor or nurse about the best option for you. Your health care team may tell you to take Senekot, Colace, Metamucil, Benefiber, or another fiber supplement containing psyllium fiber. Follow your doctor's instructions for taking a stool softener and/or laxative as prescribed.

Before starting a high-fiber diet, check with your health care team if it's appropriate for you. It may not be right for you if you are having difficulty chewing or swallowing, early fullness, loss of appetite, an intestinal blockage, or have been instructed in the past to follow a low-residue or low-fiber diet due to a medical condition.

Ways to eat and drink to manage constipation

- Adding fiber to your diet without adding enough fluids can actually make you more constipated, so drink plenty of water and other liquids per day: aim for at least 8 to 10 cups of caffeine-free liquids. Fluids to include are water; prune, pear, and other fruit juices; warm or hot drinks; decaffeinated tea and coffee, or hot water with lemon and honey. Include foods that turn to liquids at room temperature, such as ice pops, or ice cream, and foods with high water content, such as watermelon and grapes.

- Aim to eat 25 to 35 grams of fiber every day. Look at food labels and packages that boast "high fiber foods," "good source of fiber," and "more or added fiber." Look at the Nutrition Facts label for the dietary fiber per serving. Aim for cereals that contain at least 3 to 5 grams or more of fiber per serving, breads and crackers that contain at least 2 grams or more of fiber per serving, and rice and pasta that contains at least 3 grams or more of fiber per serving.

- Increase fiber gradually to prevent bloating, cramps, and gas, and be sure to drink enough fluids as you add more fiber to prevent gas and bloating. Add a glass of fluid every time you add a new high-fiber food to your day. Examples of high fiber foods are:
  - Raw and cooked fruits and vegetables (with skin, peels, and seeds). Choose raw fruit instead of fruit juice.
  - Dried fruits, such as apricots, raisins, prunes, and dates.
  - Whole-grain products: Wheat bran, whole-wheat breads and bagels; whole-grain cereals; whole-wheat pasta; whole-wheat products; whole-wheat pancakes, waffles, and muffins; and brown rice.

Be sure you see the word "whole" listed as part of the first ingredient of the product to be sure it's really a whole grain. Substitute whole-wheat flour instead of white flour in recipes.

- Nuts and seeds (sunflower, pumpkin, sesame).
- Beans (chick peas, lentils, kidney, navy, black, lima), peas, and popcorn.

- Have scheduled eating times; eat your meals and snacks at similar times every day.

- Drink warm or hot fluids, such as soup or tea, in the morning and at the beginning of meals. A great way to start your morning off is with a bowl of high-fiber bran cereal and a hot cup of coffee or tea.

- Add 1 to 2 tablespoons of ground flax seed or wheat germ to your cereal, cream of wheat, yogurt, oatmeal, or smoothies.

- Exercise helps stimulate your digestive system and keep your bowel movements regular, so talk to your doctor about a light exercise program.

- Do not wait to go to the bathroom if you feel the urge to have a bowel movement. Waiting can make constipation worse.

Foods to avoid that can worsen constipation

- High-fat dairy such as cheese, whole milk, ice cream and other dairy products.
- Foods low in fiber.
- Applesauce, bananas, white rice, white bread, and chocolate.

What can I do about uncomfortable gas and bloating?

- Limit drinks and foods that cause gas, such as carbonated drinks, broccoli, cabbage, cauliflower, cucumbers, peppers, brussels sprouts, corn, beans, peas, lentils, sauerkraut, radishes, garlic, MSG, and onions; and excessive amounts of fruit or fruit juice, such as prunes (and prune juice), apples (and apple juice), raisins (and grape juice), bananas, melons, and apricots.

- Cook your vegetables well.

- Have a small salad or fresh fruit at the end of your meal instead of eating them on an empty stomach.

- When eating "gassy" foods, try taking an over-the-counter supplement such as Beano or a similar product that contains simethicone.

- Do not use straws, and avoid chewing gum.

Fatigue

Feeling extremely tired is one of the most common, and considered one of the most distressing, side effects of cancer treatment affecting quality of life. In the medical field, it is referred to as *cancer-related fatigue*, and the key contributing factors to this are chemotherapy, radiation therapy, anemia, pain, emotional distress (depression, anxiety), sleep disturbances (insomnia), and poor diet. This type of fatigue is defined as a persistent feeling of physical, emotional, and cognitive exhaustion related to cancer treatment that interferes with normal functioning. Typically, it is more problematic with people who are undergoing more than one type of treatment, intense treatment protocols, or have advanced cancer. Because of the different possible contributing factors to fatigue, it's important that you discuss with your medical team if you are feeling fatigued and very tired, so that all of the underlying causes can be identified and treated appropriately. For most of the contributing factors, appropriate treatment and management can help reverse the issue. Some of the treatments include medications, while others include psychosocial or cognitive-behavioral treatments, such as counseling, exercise, yoga, and acupuncture.

Although it might seem intuitive to rest and avoid exercise when fatigued, research has shown significant benefits of moderate exercise in patients with cancer. People who exercise during or after the completion of treatment have much less fatigue and emotional distress, less sleep disturbances, improved functional abilities, and better quality of life when compared to those who do not exercise. Exercise programs should be individualized and take into consideration the person's medical conditions, age, gender, and type of cancer and treatment. All exercise should be started at a low level and slowly increased, as long as it remains safe to continue. For those who have limited physical mobility, you should ask for a referral to a physical therapist or ask for a rehabilitation evaluation to design a program for you. Eating and drinking well can also help you manage fatigue. If you experience fatigue that makes eating and preparing food too difficult and causes you to stop eating for more than a day, please call your doctor immediately.

? Are there any foods or drinks that can help alleviate fatigue?

Yes, you can eat and drink in a way that can help prevent fatigue. Eating enough calories and drinking enough fluids is essential to prevent fatigue. If you don't feed your body with the necessary fuels (calories and water), your body will not have enough energy to help fight against cancer.

Ways you can eat and drink to manage fatigue

- Drink plenty of caffeine-free fluids every day to prevent dehydration, which can worsen fatigue, such as water, decaf tea, 100-percent fruit juice, sports drinks (with no more than 50 calories per serving), Snapple, liquid supplements, milk, smoothies, and lemonade.

- Take a daily multivitamin to meet your basic vitamin and mineral needs. Your supplement should not be mega-doses of vitamins and should include 100 percent of the Dietary Reference Intake (DRI) of each vitamin and mineral.

- Eat five to six mini-meals and snacks each day. Always take snacks with you on the road if you leave home. When choosing which foods to eat for snacks and meals, try eating a combination of foods that contain the three nutrients that give you maximum energy: high-fiber complex carbohydrates, healthy fats, and protein. I call these "combination" meals and snacks. Some ideas include:

  - Peanut butter (protein and fat) on a piece of whole-wheat bread or with a banana (high-fiber complex carbohydrate).

  - Cheese cubes or slices (protein and fat) on crackers (high-fiber complex carbohydrates).

  - Nuts (protein and fat) with raisins (high-fiber complex carbohydrate).

  - Granola (high-fiber complex carbohydrate and fat) with yogurt or cottage cheese (protein).

  - Tuna (protein) with mayonnaise (fat) on whole-wheat bread or crackers (high-fiber complex carbohydrate).

  - Turkey slices (protein) with mayonnaise (fat) on whole-wheat roll (high-fiber complex carbohydrate).

- If you are not losing weight, avoid eating too many calories to feel energized. Gaining weight can worsen fatigue.

- Avoid large amounts of caffeine. Some caffeine is okay, but don't rely on extra caffeine to boost your energy.

- Avoid sugary drinks and desserts such as sodas, cookies, pies, and candy because high amounts of sugar can make you feel more tired.

- Avoid heavy, fatty, fried, and rich foods, which can make you feel tired.

Anemia

Anemia is a side effect of cancer and some treatments that, if untreated, can often result in fatigue. It is a condition in which you do not have enough healthy red blood cells to carry adequate oxygen to your body tissues and organs. People with anemia have low levels of hemoglobin, which is the protein inside the red blood cell that carries the oxygen. As stated earlier, there are many causes of and treatments for anemia during cancer treatment. Your doctor will evaluate the cause of your anemia with specific laboratory tests, and may prescribe medications or a blood transfusion to treat it. If you are told your anemia is related to low iron levels in your blood, there are ways to get more iron into your diet. Do not take an iron supplement unless told to do so by your doctor. Excessive iron supplementation can be harmful, leading to deposits around the heart and other organs.

Iron-rich diet

There are two types of iron in food:

- Heme iron, which comes from animal sources such as beef, poultry, pork, and fish. This type of iron is easy for your body to absorb. The darker the meat, the higher the iron content. Sources include:

- Beef, ground beef.
- Turkey (light and dark).
- Chicken breast.
- Pork loin.
- Tuna.
- Eggs.
- Non-heme iron, which comes from plant foods such as dark green vegetables and whole grains, and foods fortified with iron. Sources include:
  - Iron-fortified cereals, breads, rice, pastas. Check the Nutrition Facts panel on the food label to see that the product contains at least 20 percent or more of the Daily Value (DV) of iron.
  - Fortified instant oatmeal.
  - Beans, peas, and lentils.
  - Tofu.
  - Spinach, broccoli, kale, turnip and collard greens, potatoes with skin.
  - Raisins, dried apricots, dried figs, prunes, and prune juice.
  - Nuts and seeds.
  - Blackstrap molasses (can try 1 to 2 tablespoons on hot cereal or oatmeal).
  - Tomato sauce.

Tips to maximize iron in your diet

- Cook foods with cast-iron pots and pans.
- To better absorb non-heme iron-rich foods, eat them along with foods or drinks that contain vitamin C. For example, have a glass of orange juice (not fortified with calcium) along with fortified instant oatmeal.

- Do not eat iron-rich foods or take iron supplements with milk or calcium-rich foods. Calcium makes it harder to absorb iron. If you are taking both a calcium and iron supplement, take them at different times of the day (at least a few hours apart).

- Combine heme and non-heme iron sources at the same meal to help better absorb the non-heme iron. For example, have a roast beef sandwich with spinach and a potato.

- Do not drink coffee, tea, or soda for one hour after eating iron-rich foods or taking an iron supplement. These drinks block iron absorption.

- Do not eat iron-rich foods or take an iron supplement with high-fiber cereals.

Weight Gain

As opposed to the other side effects which can sometimes cause weight loss, there are some cancer treatments, such as some hormonal treatments, that may cause weight gain. Weight gain may also be a result of a lack of exercise and eating more food than usual as a way to cope with stress and anxiety throughout treatment. To prevent weight gain, it's important to eat the right foods, choose lower-calorie and lower-fat foods, include plenty of fiber in your diet to keep you full, and incorporate light to moderate exercise. If you have experienced more than a few pounds of weight gain, ask for a referral to a dietitian.

? What are some tips for minimizing weight gain?

Weight gain is a result of taking in more calories than you are burning. Some helpful tips for controlling an increased appetite and preventing the numbers from creeping up on the scale are:

- Do not skip meals, especially breakfast. According to the National Weight Control Registry, which provides information about what strategies work for successful weight loss and maintenance, those with successful long-term weight loss eat breakfast regularly, monitor their weight, eat consistently every day (weekdays and weekends), engage in physical activity almost every day, and eat a low-calorie, low-fat diet. To feel the fullest from breakfast, eat some protein paired with fiber (such as scrambled eggs on whole wheat toast).

- Add fiber to your diet. Eating fiber helps promote weight loss in a few ways. Firstly, it promotes satiety, which means that you feel fuller for longer after eating foods that contain fiber. This is because fiber tends to stay in your stomach longer. I like to suggest fiber-rich snacks, such as apples, to my clients working to lose weight. If you are feeling hungry, but you are not yet ready for your next meal, or you think you are about to overeat, try eating a crunchy apple. The water and fiber can help tide you over until your next meal. Secondly, high-fiber foods usually mean you have to chew more, which causes you to eat more slowly and gives your brain time to register that you are full. If you still feel hungry after the apple, you are probably ready to eat a more substantial meal. Lastly, high-fiber foods are not as calorie-dense as other foods with the same volume. One cup of green beans has far less calories than one cup of pasta. Eat more for fewer calories. Start off a meal by eating a high-fiber salad or soup, such as vegetable or lentil to help fill you up so you are less likely to overeat higher-calorie, higher-fat foods afterward.

- Drink more water and calorie-free liquids during the day to avoid mild dehydration, which is often mistaken by many for hunger. Try drinking a cup or two of water before eating food to make sure you are not mistaking hunger with thirst. Also, drink more liquids during meals. Try sparkling water, flavored seltzers, tea, coffee, and diet drinks.

- When I meet with patients, I outline with them three goals for small changes, such as adding more fruits and vegetables every day, exercising at least 30 minutes for three days per week, and eating smaller portions. Instead of feeling overwhelmed by making huge changes, thinking of doing a few things every week can help you realistically meet your goals.

- At least three-quarters of your plate should be loaded up with vegetables, fruit, whole grains, and legumes. These foods are high in fiber, vitamins, and minerals, and lower in calories and fat.

- Stop eating when you feel full. If you finish a meal and you feel like you need to unbutton or unzip your pants, chances are you ate too much at that sitting. When eating a meal, watch your portion sizes, eat slowly, and pay attention to when you are full. The quicker you eat, the more likely you are to overeat because your brain has not had enough time to recognize fullness. Before going back for seconds, make sure it's been at least 20 minutes since you finished eating so you can see if you are still hungry.

- Try to build a healthy relationship with food. Focus on adding healthy foods to your diet instead of focusing on depriving yourself of foods you shouldn't be eating. Eating healthy foods should make you feel physically and emotionally well. Instead of swearing off all high-calorie foods, you can still enjoy your favorite high-calorie foods as long as you are aware of how much you consume and you have small amounts once in a while. Try taking just a few bites of a high-calorie dish, your favorite dessert, or a few bite-size pieces of chocolate.

- Ask your doctor if you can begin to start mild to moderate exercise, such as taking a walk each day. Getting your heart rate going helps prevent weight gain, increases your energy levels, and is overall healthy for your heart. Aim for at least 30 minutes per day most days of the week. Try to keep moving by using every opportunity to add in exercise, such as walking home from work, taking the stairs, and/or taking a brisk walk at the end of the day.

- Avoid calorie-dense foods. Steer clear of high-calorie, rich desserts, such as cakes and cookies, and fast food restaurants that include many high-fat, high-calorie, and fried food options.

- When dining out, share an entrée with a friend or order an appetizer with soup or salad. If you order an entrée, before it is given to you, ask your waiter for half of it to be wrapped up to go, or try to eat only half of what's on your plate and get the rest wrapped. Also, when choosing items off of the menu, avoid foods with cream sauces, creamed and candied vegetables, gravies, and anything with the word "crispy." Go for grilled, steamed, poached, and baked choices.

- Avoid food and drinks with little nutritional value, such as high fructose corn syrup, hydrogenated or partially hydrogenated oils, sugar, and processed foods such as candies, chips, cookies, and pies. Do not waste your calories on sodas, juices, smoothies, milkshakes, and other high-calorie drinks that contain a lot of sugar and calories. When it comes to fruits, you're always better off eating the whole fruit instead of drinking a smoothie or juice because it has less calories and more fiber.

- Limit the amount of alcohol you drink, especially sweet and fruity drinks.

- Stay lean by eating plenty of lean protein sources, such as chicken (without skin), fish, beans, turkey, low-fat or nonfat cheese, skim (nonfat) or 1% milk, and egg whites.

- Do not cook when you are hungry, and try drinking water while cooking. To cut calories when cooking, use leaner cooking methods such as baking, broiling, roasting, and boiling foods; use nonstick cooking sprays instead of butter or oil; and use wine, broth, or fruit juice instead of oil.

- Try eating on a smaller plate, such as a salad plate, to watch your portion sizes.

- Keep healthy and low-calorie foods and snacks in your house so you are more likely to grab for them instead of candies, cookies, and chips. Some good ideas are reduced-fat string cheese, low-calorie yogurt, fresh fruit, and washed, bite-size pieces of raw veggies, such as carrots, celery, peppers, cucumbers, broccoli, and cauliflower.

- Be aware of your emotions when eating. Are you eating because you are actually hungry, or are you bored, tired, or stressed? If you eat for those reasons, try reaching out to a friend for support or doing something that relaxes or distracts you from eating, such as exercising, gardening, taking a walk, or taking a bath.

Chapter 5

Menus and Recipes for Treatment

The last thing you want to worry about during treatment is food preparation, cooking, and menu planning. Whether you are feeling nauseated or experiencing bouts of diarrhea, you want to eat food that is easy to prepare, gives you comfort, and makes you feel better physically and emotionally. In times of sickness, such as having the flu or a cold, you want to feel comforted by the food you are eating, and avoid too much hassle by cooking. For those of you experiencing symptoms during treatment, it's important that you eat and cook foods that make you feel better, not worse. Foods that give you comfort in times of sadness, sickness, and also at happy occasions, are referred to as "comfort foods." According to the American Institute for Cancer Research (AICR), "comfort foods can be defined as feel-good, hearty foods that are both nourishing and nurturing." Comfort foods remind you of your past with their textures, smells, and tastes. For the most part, these foods are creamy, soft, rich, and warm and contain a lot of fat. Think macaroni and cheese, chicken soup, mashed potatoes, pizza, and meatloaf.

The menus listed here are to help give you ideas on how to make high-calorie, high-protein meals for those of you struggling to keep your weight stable. If it's too difficult to make your own meals, ask friends or family if they can help. You can also cook larger amounts of food on the days that you feel better, and freeze extra portions for later. If needed, you can also buy ready-made meals from the supermarket. If you are lactose intolerant, substitute regular cow's milk with LactAid milk, rice milk, almond milk, or soy milk. For additional calories, try the sweetened versions. Also, take LactAid pills when you eat other dairy foods, such as ice cream. You will notice that fruits and vegetables are not major components of the menus provided. While they do contain plenty of healthy nutrients that are recommended for cancer prevention, they are low in calories and should not be the focus of your diet right now if weight loss is your issue.

Menu Ideas

The following menus can help you plan high-calorie, high-protein meals and snacks along with the tips listed in Chapter 4. Aim to separate meals and snacks by two to three hours.

Meal or Snack	Day 1	Day 2	Day 3
Breakfast	1 scrambled egg omelet (2 eggs scrambled with a few splashes of whole milk or 1 container of Benecalorie supplement) topped with 1 ounce of your favorite shredded cheese. Melt 1 - 2 teaspoons of butter in the pan. 1/2 English muffin or 1 slice of toast, buttered 1/2 cup of your favorite 100% juice	2 pancakes, waffles, or slices of French toast topped with butter and maple syrup 1 hard-boiled egg 1/2 cup of your favorite 100% juice or fruit nectar	1 cup of oatmeal prepared with double strength milk or vanilla liquid supplement, butter, sugar/brown sugar, a sprinkle of nuts and raisins (do not add sugar if you use the vanilla liquid supplement) 1/2 cup 100% juice, or fruit nectar, or double strength milk
Snack	1/2 cup of trail mix (nuts and dried fruits) 1/2 cup of juice, liquid supplement, or homemade shake or smoothie	1 cup homemade shake or smoothie or 1/3 cup of granola mixed into 1 cup of fruit yogurt with 1/2 cup of fruit nectar	1/2 cup of 4% cottage cheese mixed with your favorite jam topped on crackers 1/2 cup of double strength milk, liquid supplement or homemade shake

Lunch	1/2 cup of macaroni and cheese topped with extra grated cheese 1/2 cup of peas with butter 1/2 cup of double strength milk or fruit nectar	1/2 sandwich of turkey and cheese on your favorite bread or roll (save the other 1/2 of the sandwich for another snack or meal) 1/2 cup of chocolate milk or fruit nectar	1/2 of a sandwich with tuna salad, chicken salad, or egg salad (made with regular mayonnaise) 1/2 cup of 100% fruit juice or fruit nectar
Snack	2 tablespoons of peanut butter on your favorite crackers 1/2 cup milk, liquid supplement, or shake	1–2 ounces of your favorite (melted) cheese or 4 tablespoons of hummus on top of 1 slice of bread, half a pita, or half a bagel 1/2 cup of fruit nectar or 100% fruit juice	2 handfuls of your favorite nuts 1/2 cup of your favorite dried fruit 1/2 cup of juice, milk, or milkshake
Dinner	1 (2-inch) slice of lasagna or quiche 1/2 cup of cooked cauliflower with bread crumbs sautéed in butter or oil 1/2 cup of 100% fruit juice or smoothie	3 ounces of steak or fried chicken 1/2 cup of creamed corn 1/2 cup mashed potatoes prepared with butter, double strength milk or cream, topped with gravy or cheese	1 cup of baked ziti prepared with whole-milk ricotta and mozzarella cheese 1/2 cup of green beans almondine 1/2 cup of double strength milk (pg. 140) or milkshake
Snack	1/2 cup of ice cream topped with your favorite nuts, syrup, and whipped cream	1 8-ounce container of fruit yogurt (regular or Greek yogurt)	1/2 cup of custard or rice pudding topped with whipped cream

Snack ideas to add calories and protein

- 1 cup of pasta, 2 slices of American cheese, and 1/2 cup of whole milk
- 2 ounces of meat, 2 slices of bread, 2 tsp. mayonnaise
- 2 waffles or pancakes, 1 Tbsp. butter, 4 Tbsp. syrup
- 1 ounce of pretzels, 1/4 cup nuts, 1/4 cup raisins (or 1 small box) or dried cranberries
- 1 cup 4% cottage cheese, 1/2 cup fruit or 1 cup canned fruit
- 1 bagel, 2 Tbsp. cream cheese, 2 Tbsp. jam or jelly
- 2 slices of bread, 2 Tbsp. peanut butter, 2 Tbsp. jelly
- 1 banana, 1/2 cup sour cream
- 1 banana, 1 Tbsp. honey, 1 Tbsp. peanut butter
- 2 Tbsp. hummus, 1 pita
- 1 apple, 2 Tbsp. peanut butter, almond butter, or cashew butter
- 1 cup of veggies, 4 Tbsp. salad dressing
- 4 wafers, 3/4 cup of milk
- 1 tortilla, 3/4 cup beans, 1/4 cup of shredded cheese
- 1 cup of regular yogurt (or Greek yogurt), 1/4 cup granola, 1/2 cup berries
- 3 Tbsp. trail mix, 1 ounce of cheese
- 1/2 cup creamed soup, 8 saltines
- 1/4 avocado, 1 pita
- 1 small baked potato, 1 Tbsp. butter, 1/4 cup shredded cheese
- 1 cup dry cereal, 1 cup milk
- 1 English muffin, 2 scrambled eggs, 1 Tbsp. butter

Recipes During Treatment

The recipes in this chapter are organized by symptoms. The majority of these recipes are higher in calories, protein, and fat to help prevent weight loss that is commonly seen during treatment. For those of you who are not experiencing weight loss, you should focus on cutting back on some of the higher-calorie additions to these recipes, for example: substitute whole fat and full-fat ingredients with their reduced-fat or fat-free versions. Follow the suggestions listed in Chapter 7. My goal is that you or your caregiver can use these easy-to-prepare and hassle-free recipes to fit your specific needs during treatment. For each of the side effects listed here, you can refer back to Chapter 4 for detailed suggestions for managing symptoms.

Nausea

Chicken Soup
Yield: 8-10 servings.

1 (3- to 5- pound) chicken, quartered

12 cups water

3 carrots

1 stalk celery

2 parsnips

1 onion

1 Tbsp. salt

1/4 tsp. pepper

1 sweet potato, diced

1 zucchini, sliced

Optional Ingredients:

Few sprigs of fresh dill

1 parsley root, chopped

1 garlic clove, peeled (pierce with toothpick in order to remove easily after cooking)

1. Clean chicken and remove excess fat.

2. Fill an 8-quart pot with 12 cups of water, chicken, and vegetables.

3. Bring mixture to a boil, skimming residue from top.

4. Add salt and pepper. If using optional ingredients, add chopped parsley root, dill, and garlic.

5. Reduce heat and simmer covered for about 2 hours. Remove garlic clove before serving.

6. To remove excess fat, prepare soup in advance and refrigerate for several hours or overnight. Fat will congeal on top. Remove and heat soup before serving.

Per serving: 184 calories, 8 g protein, 7 g fat, 23 g carbohydrate, 4 g fiber, 953 mg sodium, 24 mg cholesterol

Best Matzoh Balls

These matzoh balls bring heartiness and comfort to any chicken soup. They can be eaten alone as a snack or as a side dish with some gravy. You can also freeze (covered) matzo balls for later use.

Yield: About 18 matzoh balls

1 cup matzoh meal

4 large eggs, lightly beaten

1/4 cup canola or light vegetable oil

1/4 cup water

2 tsp. salt

1. Combine matzoh meal, eggs, oil, water, and salt in a medium bowl and mix with a fork until dry ingredients are moistened and there are no lumps.

2. Cover and refrigerate for 30 minutes.

3. Bring a large pot of salted water to a rolling boil. Wet hands lightly with water and remove heaping tablespoons of the matzoh mixture and roll into 1–2 inch balls and drop into the pot of boiling water.

4. Let it boil until all matzoh balls float to the top, then cover tightly and reduce heat to a low boil (rolling simmer) for 40 minutes. When the balls fluff, remove them with a slotted spoon and serve with soup.

Per serving: 68 calories, 2 g protein, 4 g fat, 5 g carbohydrate, 0.1 g fiber, 16 mg sodium, 47 m g cholesterol

Soothing Ginger Tea

Ginger can help calm your stomach and decrease nausea. According to a recent study funded by the National Cancer Institute, ginger helped prevent or reduce chemotherapy-induced nausea when taken with traditional anti-nausea drugs for six days (three days before chemotherapy, the day of chemotherapy, and the two days after chemotherapy). The most effective doses were 1/4 to 1/2 of a teaspoon of ginger each day. You can use fresh or dry ginger. Ginger flavored foods and drinks, such as ginger snaps, ginger ale, dried ginger, and crystallized ginger, can also be helpful. Talk to your doctor before taking ginger because it has the potential to interfere with blood clotting and prolong bleeding time.

Yield: 1 cup

1 cup of water

1-inch piece of fresh ginger root

1 tablespoon of honey

Lemon slice or 1 tablespoon lemon juice (optional)

1. Peel the ginger root and finely mince it or thinly slice it.

2. Boil the water in a saucepan. Once the water is boiling, add the ginger root to the saucepan.

3. Cover and reduce to a simmer for 15–20 minutes. Strain out the ginger root and keep the liquid tea.

4. Add honey and lemon to taste. Slowly sip the tea between meals and snacks or with meals to soothe your stomach.

Per serving: 76 calories, 0 g protein, 0 g fat, 20 g carbohydrate, 0 g fiber, 5 mg sodium, 0 mg cholesterol

Carrot-Ginger Muffins

Muffins are a great idea to use as a singe-serving snack that you can bring to your treatment. After making a batch of muffins, you can freeze them until you are ready to use them. They are mildly spiced, easy on your stomach, and have a little ginger to add flavor and help relieve nausea.

Yield: 12 muffins

8 ounces jarred baby food carrots

2 eggs

3/4 cup sugar

1 cup flour

1/2 cup oil

1/2 tsp. salt

1/2 tsp. baking powder

1/2 tsp. baking soda

1 tsp. vanilla

1/2 tsp. cinnamon

1/4 tsp. ground ginger

1. Preheat oven to 350 degrees.

2. Grease 12 muffin tins with nonstick cooking spray.

3. In a large mixing bowl, combine all ingredients and mix well. If using an electric stand mixer, beat at medium speed until the batter is smooth.

4. Pour the batter into prepared tins. Bake, uncovered, for 15 minutes or until a toothpick inserted into the center of one of the muffins comes out dry.

Per serving: 186 calories, 2 g protein, 10 g fat, 22 g carbohydrate, 1 g fiber, 131 mg sodium, 35 mg cholesterol

Diarrhea

Banana Oatmeal

This is a great warm and creamy mini-meal or breakfast that is low-fat and contains binding soluble fiber (from the oatmeal and bananas) to help thicken your stool. If regular milk bothers your stomach, substitute it with lactose-free milk such as soy milk or Lactaid milk.

Yield: 4 servings

3 cups of skim milk

3 Tbsp. brown sugar

2 cups oatmeal

1 cup sliced bananas

1. Bring milk, brown sugar, and oatmeal to a boil over medium-high heat.

2. Stir in oatmeal. Cook for 5 minutes or until all the liquid is absorbed.

3. Remove from stove. Pour into small bowl and top with sliced bananas.

Per serving: 275 calories, 12 g protein, 3 g fat, 52 g carbohydrate, 5 g fiber, 82 mg sodium, 4 mg cholesterol

Oatmeal Pancakes

You can enjoy these pancakes at home or pack a few with you as a snack when you are away from home. You can also eat these pancakes with applesauce for additional binding power. If you're eating these on the road, pack a single-serving applesauce. This recipe is also a good choice for people with sore or dry mouth, if you moisten the pancakes by melting some butter and soaking them with maple syrup.

Yield: Approximately 8 pancakes

1/2 cup all purpose flour

1/2 cup quick-cooking or old-fashioned oatmeal

1/2 cup skim milk (substitute with lactose-free milk, such as soy milk or Lactaid milk if regular milk bothers your stomach)

1 tsp. baking powder

1/2 tsp. baking soda

1/4 tsp. salt

1/4 cup sugar

1/2 cup unsweetened applesauce

2 large egg whites

1 Tbsp. canola oil

1. In a medium bowl, combine all ingredients and whisk until well-blended.

2. Heat griddle or skillet over medium heat or to 375 degrees. When the skillet is hot, pour about 1/4 cup of pancake batter per pancake.

3. Cook until bubbles appear and edges have puffed. Flip the pancakes and cook until golden.

4. Eat with warmed applesauce and a sprinkle of cinnamon, and drizzle some maple syrup on top of pancakes.

Per serving: 129 calories, 9 g protein, 2 g protein, 19 g carbohydrate, 1 g fiber, 319 mg sodium, 0 mg cholesterol

Constipation

Hearty Meat and Veggie Soup

Flavorful and packed with fiber, this soup is more like a meal in a bowl. Do not forget to eat high-fiber meals along with a cup of water to relieve constipation.

Yields: 8–10 servings

1 Tbsp. oil

1 onion, diced

2 cloves garlic, minced

1 pound stew meat, cut into 1-inch cubes

9 cups water

1 1/2 tsp. salt

1/4 tsp. pepper

1/3 cup barley

1/2 cup lima beans

1 cup split peas

1 bay leaf

1 potato, diced

2 large carrots, sliced

2 celery stalks, diced

1 cup fresh string beans, chopped

1 (16-ounce) can tomato sauce

2 Tbsp. parsley, chopped

1. Heat oil and sauté onion and garlic in 6-quart pot for about 2 minutes.

2. Add stew meat, water, salt, pepper, barley, split peas, and bay leaf.

3. Bring to a boil, then lower flame and simmer, covered for 1 hour.

4. Add potato, carrots, celery, string beans, tomato sauce, and parsley, and cook for another 1 1/2 hours. Serve hot.

Per Serving: 300 calories, 18 g protein, 10 g fat, 36 g carbohydrate, 10 g fiber, 661 mg sodium, 30 mg cholesterol

Sautéed Vegetable Salad

This salad is a beautiful combination of colors, filled with healthy antioxidants, is quick and easy to prepare, and has a delicious flavor. The wide array of vegetables with their skins, along with the beans, really packs in the fiber. Adding lentils adds even more fiber.

Yield: 8–10 servings

1 eggplant, unpeeled, cut into 3/4-inch dice

1 yellow squash with skin, cut into 1/2-inch dice

1 zucchini with skin, cut into 1/2-inch dice

3 Portobello mushroom caps cut into 1/2-inch dice

½ red onion cut into 1/4-inch dice

1 red bell pepper, seeded, cut into 1/2-inch dice

Fine sea salt and ground black pepper

1 (15-ounce) can chickpeas (garbanzo beans), drained and rinsed

1 (15-ounce) can lentils, drained and rinsed (optional)

Dressing:

1/4 cup balsamic vinegar

1/2 cup extra-virgin olive oil

1 (1-ounce) packet Good Seasons Italian Dressing mix

1. Place all diced vegetables into a large bowl.

2. Combine balsamic vinegar, oil, and seasoning packet in a jar or cruet and shake or whisk to blend. Pour dressing over vegetables.

3. Heat 1 Tbsp. olive oil in large skillet over medium heat. Add the vegetables and sauté until shiny and softened, 5-6 minutes. Remove from heat. Transfer to a large bowl.

4. Add chickpeas and lentils (optional). Serve warm or at room temperature.

Per serving (with lentils): 240 calories, 7 g protein, 12 g fat, 28 g carbohydrate, 8 g fiber, 480 mg sodium, 0 mg cholesterol

Sore mouth and throat and dry mouth

Myrna's Macaroni and Cheese
I grew up on this meal, and all my friends looked forward to coming over for this soupy macaroni and cheese. Unlike other macaroni and cheese recipes, this makes a milky, soupy dish that is better when eaten with a spoon! This is a great recipe for those who have difficulty chewing or swallowing and for those with dry mouth who need well-moistened foods. It also is quick and easy and does not require baking time. Not only does this have calories and protein, but it's a good source of calcium.

Yield: 4 servings

2 cups elbow macaroni

1 cup whole milk

7 slices American cheese

2 Tbsp. butter

Dash of salt and pepper

1. Cook noodles according to package directions; drain, stir in the butter until melted, and set aside.

2. Pour milk into large microwaveable bowl. Using your hands, tear each slice of cheese into smaller pieces (about 4 pieces per slice) and add to milk.

3. Cover and microwave for 7 minutes on 50 percent power.

4. Stir cheese sauce until all the cheese is completely mixed in and the mixture is smooth. If cheese is clumpy, microwave for 1 additional minute. Add noodles to cheese sauce and mix well. Add salt and pepper to taste.

Per serving: 370 calories, 16 g protein, 24 g fat, 23 g carbohydrate, 0.9 g fiber, 775 mg sodium, 68 mg cholesterol

 ## Creamy Corn Soufflé

This soufflé is creamy, sweet, and very soft. It is almost a pudding consistency, and makes a great side dish.

Yield: 12–14 servings

2 (15-ounce) cans creamed-style corn

1/4 cup sugar

1/2 cup (1 stick) margarine or butter, melted

3 large eggs

1/2 cup flour

1 tsp. baking powder

3/4 cup milk

1/4 cup water

1 tsp. vanilla

1. Preheat oven to 350 degrees.

2. In a large bowl, mix the corn, sugar, margarine, eggs, flour, baking powder, milk, water, and vanilla.

3. Pour into a lightly greased 9-x-13-inch baking dish

4. Bake, uncovered for 1 1/2 hours.

Per Serving: 220 calories, 4 g protein, 9 g fat, 24 g carbohydrate, 1 g fiber, 272 mg sodium, 50 mg cholesterol

Challah Bread French Toast Soufflé

This is a mouth-watering, very rich, and creamy version of French toast that can be enjoyed as a high-calorie and high-protein snack or mini-meal all week long. Everyone who has tried this recipe says it's the best French toast they've ever eaten. I agree.

Yield: 8–10 servings

1/2 cup unsalted butter

1 cup dark brown sugar, firmly packed

2 Tbsp. light corn syrup

6 (1-inch thick) sliced challah bread, crust removed

5 large eggs

1 1/2 cups half-and-half

1 tsp. vanilla extract

1/4 tsp. salt

1. Preheat oven to 350 degrees.

2. In a heavy saucepan, combine butter, brown sugar, and corn syrup over medium heat. Stir occasionally until melted and smooth. Pour mixture into 9-x-13-inch baking dish.

3. Trim crusts from the bead and arrange in one layer in the baking dish.

4. In a large mixing bowl, whisk together eggs, half-and-half, vanilla, and salt, and pour evenly over the bread.

5. Bake, uncovered for 35–40 minutes or until puffed and edges are light golden brown. Serve with pieces turned over and caramel on top.

Per serving: 343 calories, 7 g protein, 17.8 g fat, 39 g carbohydrate, 0.3 g fiber, 228 mg sodium, 146 mg cholesterol

Taste and smell changes

Sweet and Sour Meatballs

If meat tastes strange to you, these meatballs have a sweet-and-sour flavor that may help mask that. To make this a complete meal, top cooked rice with meatballs.

Yield: 24 meatballs

1 pound ground beef

1 egg, beaten

1/2 cup bread crumbs

1/2 onion, grated

3/4 tsp. pepper

1/2 tsp. oregano

Sauce:

1 cup jellied cranberry sauce

3/4 cup ketchup

1/4 cup brown sugar

2 tsp. lemon juice

1. In a large mixing bowl, combine ground beef, egg, bread crumbs, onion, and seasonings.

2. Form meat into 1-inch balls.

3. In a 3-quart saucepan, combine cranberry sauce, ketchup, brown sugar, and lemon juice. Cook over low flame for 25–30 minutes, stirring often.

4. Add meatballs to sauce and simmer for 1 hour.

5. Serve with hot, cooked rice.

Per Serving: 86 calories, 4 g protein, 3 g fat, 11 g carbohydrate, 0 g fiber, 119 mg sodium, 22 mg cholesterol

Sesame Noodles

This recipe has a combination of flavor-enhancing ingredients like garlic, tahini, soy sauce, chili sauce, and red wine vinegar. I've tried many varieties of sesame noodle recipes, but this recipe has the most delicious flavor and a creamy consistency that can awaken your taste buds.

Yield: 8 servings

1 (16-ounce) package linguine noodles, cooked

1 Tbsp. sesame oil

1 medium cucumber, peeled and chopped

3 scallions, chopped

2 tsp. sesame seeds

Sauce:

1/2 cup peanut oil

2 tsp. garlic

4 ounces sesame paste (tahini)

1 Tbsp. chili sauce (or Chinese hot sauce)

6 Tbsp. soy sauce

6 Tbsp. red wine vinegar

4 Tbsp. sugar

1 tsp. salt

1. Cook linguine according to package directions; drain and transfer to a large serving bowl.

2. Mix linguine with sesame oil and refrigerate to chill.

3. In a medium bowl, mix all ingredients for sauce together. Pour over linguine, tossing to coat.

4. Garnish with sesame seeds, scallions, and cucumbers.

Per Serving: 472 calories, 12 g protein, 24 g fat, 53 g carbohydrate, 4 g fiber, 790 mg sodium, 0 mg cholesterol

Weight gain

Low calorie recipes

These recipes are lighter and lower in calories than the other recipes in this book. They are intended for those struggling with weight gain during treatment, and for cancer survivors who completed treatment and maintain a healthy weight. Enjoy these veggie dishes with lean proteins, such as turkey, chicken, or fish.

Crunchy Corn Salad

This salad is not only tasty, crunchy, and packed with fiber, but it's also quick and easy!

Yield: 8 servings

2 (15-ounce) cans yellow corn, drained

1 (7-ounce) can white corn, drained

1 small red onion, diced

1 red bell pepper, diced

8 ounces snow peas, sliced into small pieces

3 Tbsp. olive oil

Salt to taste

Pepper to taste

1. Mix ingredients together. Add salt and pepper to taste.

Per Serving: 166 calories, 4 g protein, 6 g fat, 29 g carbohydrate, 4 g fiber, 358 mg sodium, 0 mg cholesterol

Edamame Salad

This is a light salad that is not drenched in oil as other salad recipes are. The edamame adds protein and fiber, making it more filling, and the soy nuts add a little crunch to this salad. You can buy either fresh shelled edamame, or buy them frozen and cook them for 5 minutes in boiling (salted) water. Drain, run cold water over them, and then pat dry.

Yield: 6 servings

5 leaves Romaine lettuce, shredded

4 ounces mesculun or spring mix lettuces

1 1/2 cups (8 ounces) shelled edamame

1 cup grape tomatoes, halved

1/4 tsp. coarse sea salt

1/4 cup extra-virgin olive oil

2 Tbsp. balsamic vinegar

1/4 tsp. cayenne pepper

1/4 tsp. ground black pepper

Handful of roasted and salted soybeans (soy nuts)

1. In a large salad bowl, add the lettuce, edamame, and tomato halves and sprinkle with the sea salt

2. In a jar or container, add olive oil, balsamic vinegar, cayenne pepper, and black pepper. Whisk or shake the ingredients until well-blended.

3. Pour the dressing over the salad and toss to mix. Sprinkle the soy nuts on top.

Per serving: 164 calories, 7 g protein, 12 g fat, 9 g carbohydrate, 3 g fiber, 109 mg sodium, 0 mg cholesterol

Weight loss

High calorie recipes

Tuna Casserole

This tuna casserole contains a combination of carbohydrates, protein and fat.

Yield: 6–8 servings

2 cups elbow macaroni

1 can condensed cream of mushroom soup

1 large can French's french fried onions

1 cup whole milk

2 (5-ounce) cans tuna (chunk light), drained

1. Preheat oven to 350 degrees.

2. Cook the pasta according to package directions; drain and place in a large serving bowl.

3. Spray a 9-x-13-inch pan with nonstick cooking spray.

4. Mix pasta with remaining ingredients, pour into the pan, and bake for 45 minutes.

Per Serving: 378 calories, 18 g protein, 17 g fat, 37 g carbohydrate, 1 g fiber, 659 mg sodium, 18 mg cholesterol

Soft Scalloped Potatoes

If you're looking to try a variation of potatoes other than mashed potatoes or baked potatoes, this recipe makes 10–12 servings of a creamy potato side dish that you can enjoy throughout the week. These potatoes are calorie-packed, soft, creamy, mild, and easy to chew and swallow for those with a sore or dry mouth.

Yield: 10–12 servings

2 Tbsp. margarine

3 Tbsp. oil

1/2 cup flour

2 large onions, chopped (omit if mouth sores present)

1/2 cup mayonnaise

1–2 tsp. salt

24 ounces chicken broth

8 large Idaho potatoes, peeled and sliced into 1/4-inch slices

Black pepper

Paprika

1. Preheat oven to 350 degrees.

2. Spray a 9-x-13-inch glass or ceramic baking dish with non-stick cooking spray.

3. In a large pot, melt the margarine and oil over medium-high heat. Add the flour, stirring constantly. Add the onions, mayonnaise, salt, and chicken broth. Stir until smooth. Cook until the sauce thickens.

4. Using a ladle, place a layer of the sauce on the bottom of the prepared pan. Spread a layer of overlapping potatoes. Top with a layer of sauce. Repeat, alternating with layers of potatoes and sauce two more times.

5. There should be a total of three sauce layers and two potato layers, with sauce on top. Sprinkle the top layer with pepper (omit if mouth sores present) and paprika. Bake uncovered for 1 1/2 hours or until golden.

Per Serving: 234 calories, 3 g protein, 10 g fat, 34 g carbohydrate, 2 g fiber, 511 mg sodium, 5 mg cholesterol

High protein recipes

Egg Salad

Egg salad is a soft, easy-to-chew and swallow food that is a great source of protein and calories. You can eat this alone, on a sandwich, or on top of crackers. This recipe is great for someone with dry mouth, too.

Yield: 4 servings

7 hard-boiled eggs

1/2 Tbsp. oil

1 medium onion, chopped (optional)

1 celery stalk, finely chopped

2 Tbsp. mayonnaise

1/2 tsp. prepared mustard

Dash of pepper

1. Peel hard-boiled eggs and mash in a medium bowl with oil and salt.

2. Add onion, celery, and mayonnaise, and mix well with mustard and pepper.

Per serving: 193 calories, 12 g protein, 14 g fat, 6 g carbohydrate, 1 g fiber, 181 mg sodium, 373 mg cholesterol

Spinach quiche

Quiches are soft and easy-to-chew, and made up of protein-rich ingredients: eggs, cheese, and milk. A slice of quiche can be eaten alone as a mini-meal or along with a side dish as part of a meal. This is another recipe that someone with sore or dry mouth can enjoy.

Yield: 9 servings

2 large eggs, lighty beaten

1/2 cup whole milk

1/2 cup mayonnaise

1 small onion, chopped (omit with mouth sores)

1 (10-ounce) package frozen chopped spinach, thawed and drained

4 tablespoons flour

2 cups (8 ounces) shredded cheddar cheese

2 cups (8 ounces) shredded mozzarella cheese

1. Preheat oven to 350 degrees.

2. In a large bowl, combine eggs, milk, mayonnaise, onion, spinach, flour, and cheddar cheese.

3. Pour into a greased 9-inch or 8-x-8-inch baking dish. Sprinkle with mozzarella.

4. Bake for 30–45 minutes or until puffed the center and knife inserted in the center come out clean.

Per Serving: 275 calories, 15 g protein, 20 g fat, 9 g carbohydrate, 1 g fiber, 450 mg sodium, 98 mg cholesterol

Energy-Boosting, High-Protein Milkshakes and Smoothies

Homemade milkshakes and smoothies are very useful when you have difficulty swallowing, taste changes, poor appetite, or weight loss. When made with the most energy-boosting, protein-rich ingredients, these shakes pack in calories and protein in just one glass. The following recipes can be modified according to your taste buds. Be creative and experiment with various ingredients that add calories and flavor. **Caution: *Never* add raw eggs to your shakes; raw eggs may cause salmonella food poisoning.** Only use fresh fruit if your medical team allows it. When using fresh fruit, wash it before using in a smoothie.

Non-fat dry milk powder is one of my favorite protein supplements. It is made of whey protein, can be found in any supermarket, and is less expensive when compared to other protein supplements sold at popular nutrition stores. The powder can be mixed into soups, scrambled eggs, cereal, sauces, gravies, and mashed potatoes, as well as into smoothie and shake recipes to add calories and protein. You can also use the powder to make double strength milk, which contains 40 percent more calories and twice the protein per serving of regular milk, and use in place of regular milk in any recipe or drink it by itself.

For the following recipes, place all ingredients in a blender or use a hand-held blender. Blend on high speed until smooth. Add additional liquid if you would like to make your shake thinner. Chill the drink before serving. Most of these recipes make a few glasses, so store unused drinks in the refrigerator (for no more than one day) or freezer, and blend it again later with a few ice cubes or a little more liquid. A serving is based on your preference; it can be a 1/2 to 1 cup for a snack, or more than that if you use the drink to substitute for a meal.

For maximum calories and protein, use the plus varieties of liquid supplements in recipes (Boost Plus, Ensure Plus). To make any of these recipes lactose-free, substitute regular milk with soy, rice, almond, oat, or Lactaid milk, and use soy ice cream instead of regular ice cream.

Double Strength Milk
Yield: 4 servings

1 quart of whole milk

1 envelope of non-fat dry milk powder (buy at any supermarket)

Pour liquid milk into a deep bowl and add the dry milk powder. With a mixer or hand mixer, blend until the dry milk fully dissolves and refrigerate.

Per Serving: 228 calories, 16 g protein, 8 g fat, 25 g carbohydrate, 0 g fiber, 222 mg sodium, 28 mg cholesterol

Basic Liquid Supplement Milkshake
Yield: 3 servings

1 cup of whole milk or double strength milk

1 cup of premium ice cream (any flavor)

1 can of commercial liquid supplement

Per serving (when using "plus" variety of liquid supplement and double strength milk): 372 calories, 12 g protein, 18 g fat, 41 g carbohydrate, 0 g fiber, 197 mg sodium, 77 mg cholesterol

Iced Mocha Latte
Yield: 1 serving

1 can of any commercial liquid supplement (use "plus" for more calories and protein)

2 tsp. instant coffee (can use flavored like hazelnut or vanilla)

2 tsp. chocolate syrup

1/2 cup ice cubes

Per serving (when using "plus" variety of liquid supplement): 404 calories, 14 g protein, 13 g fat, 59 g carbohydrate, 0 g fiber, 284 mg sodium, 5 mg cholesterol

Frozen Hot Chocolate
Yield: 2 servings

1 cup premium vanilla ice cream

1/2 cup whole milk or liquid supplement

1 envelope of regular hot chocolate mix

1/2 cup ice cubes

Top with whipped cream (optional)

Per serving (with whipped cream and "plus" liquid supplement): 450 calories, 8 g protein, 24 g fat, 50 g carbohydrate, 1 g fiber, 215 mg sodium, 111 mg cholesterol

Berry Smoothie
(Skip this recipe if you have diarrhea because of the high fiber content and skip it if you have a sore mouth because the berries and flaxseeds may irritate your mouth.)

Yield: 1 serving

1 cup fresh or frozen mixed berries (or any berry of your choice, i.e., raspberry, blueberry, strawberry)

½ cup plain or vanilla yogurt

1 medium banana, peeled

1 Tbsp. ground flax seeds or wheat germ (optional)

1 cup whole milk or liquid supplement

Per serving (using "plus" liquid supplement and vanilla yogurt): 679 calories, 23 g protein, 116 carbohydrate, 10 g fiber, 328 mg sodium, 11 mg cholesterol

High-Calorie Pudding
Yield: 2 servings

1 can liquid supplement

1 (3.4 ounce) package instant pudding mix

Add liquid supplement to the pudding mix. Blend with a wire whisk for 2 minutes and refrigerate until it sets.

Per serving: 364 calories, 7 g protein, 6 g fat, 71 g carbohydrate, 0 g fiber, 833 mg sodium, 3 mg cholesterol

Chapter 6

Navigating the Supermarket

There are two things that commonly happen to me when grocery shopping: one, if I'm hungry at the time, I will undoubtedly pick things off the shelves that I did not plan to buy; and two, I grab more products off the shelves if I did not come in with a shopping list. Supermarkets are designed to maximize your spending while shopping, and food products are cleverly advertised to push the buying power even further. Nothing is accidental in the supermarket, and products are placed on specific shelves at specific levels to make the shopper likely to purchase more food than originally intended. For this reason, I counsel my patients who are following a healthy diet to shop smarter. Sit down for a few minutes before you go to the supermarket, make a shopping list, and don't go to the supermarket when you're starving! For those looking to maintain or lose weight, follow the rule of planning ahead and avoid impulsive unhealthy purchases. For those experiencing a loss of appetite and weight loss during or after treatment, you also should make a shopping list before you go; however, you should actually go food shopping when you are hungry, so you may be more enticed to pick up foods that you see. Walking through the supermarket aisles and seeing food in front of you may trigger your appetite and give you ideas for snacks and meals when your appetite is not giving you ideas. Writing a shopping list beforehand with some of the suggestions listed on the following pages can also guide you on what to stock up on to maximize your diet.

Grocery List for Before and During Treatment

The majority of this grocery list consists of food items that are high calorie to prevent weight loss. It also lists a wide range of food staples that you can choose from based on your symptoms(s) during treatment. To choose the best products for your kitchen, base it on your symptom(s), and follow the diet recommendations for symptom control in Chapter 4. Also, choose items from this list that you know you like and use most often. If you are not up to doing your own grocery shopping, ask friends and family to go the store for you with a list of the foods that you check off below. Note: If weight loss is not an issue, you can use this list, but choose whole-grains, leaner meats, and lower-fat varieties of the items listed. You can use the suggestions for a plant-based diet in Chapter 7 to help guide your choices.

Bread/grains

Note: for those with constipation, choose whole grain products; for those with diarrhea, choose white products.

- ☐ White or whole-wheat bread, English muffins, bagels, dinner rolls, pita bread
- ☐ Pizza crusts, focaccia bread
- ☐ Pasta, noodles
- ☐ Rice (white, brown, quick cooking)
- ☐ Oatmeal
- ☐ Farina
- ☐ Cream of Wheat or Cream of Rice

- ❑ Grits
- ❑ Granola
- ❑ Your favorite cereals
- ❑ Bread crumbs
- ❑ Couscous
- ❑ Barley
- ❑ Matzoh
- ❑ Rice cakes

Dairy/Milk:

- ❑ Yogurt (whole, sweetened) or Greek yogurt
- ❑ Milk (whole or 2%)
- ❑ Evaporated milk (can be used instead of water when cooking)
- ❑ Sweetened condensed milk
- ❑ Cheese (varieties)
- ❑ Shredded cheese
- ❑ Ice cream or frozen yogurt
- ❑ 4% cottage cheese
- ❑ Cream cheese
- ❑ Sour cream
- ❑ Half-and-half, heavy cream

Meat, poultry, legumes, fish, and eggs

- ❑ Beef (ground, roast)
- ❑ Chicken
- ❑ Turkey, ground
- ❑ Tofu (pasteurized; soft, silken or firm)
- ❑ Pork
- ❑ Shrimp

- Eggs
- Pasteurized egg products (i.e., Egg Beaters)
- Lentils
- Beans (canned): black, pinto, kidney, garbanzo (chickpeas), refried
- Salmon (fresh or canned)
- Tuna (fresh or canned)
- Mackerel, herring, sardines, trout, red snapper, cod, flounder, sole
- Hummus
- Soybeans, edamame

Fats and oils

- Olive, canola, almond, or peanut oil
- Mayonnaise
- Butter or margarine
- Gravy
- Ground flax seeds or flax seed oil
- Olives

Nuts and seeds

- Nuts (pecans, macadamia, brazil, walnuts, almonds, peanuts)
- Seeds (sunflower, pumpkin)
- Nut butters (peanut butter, almond butter, cashew butter); peanut butter in single-serving packages

Fruit (fresh, canned, or dried)

- Frozen or fresh berries (raspberries, strawberries, blueberries, blackberries)
- Bananas

- ❑ Pears
- ❑ Papayas
- ❑ Peachs
- ❑ Nectarines
- ❑ Watermelons
- ❑ Lemon, limes
- ❑ Melons
- ❑ Apples
- ❑ Mangoes
- ❑ Avocados
- ❑ Dried fruits (raisins, dried cranberries, figs, dates, prunes, papaya, ginger, apples, pears, apricots)

Vegetables (fresh, frozen, or canned)

- ❑ Broccoli
- ❑ Cauliflower
- ❑ Green beans
- ❑ Spinach
- ❑ Peas
- ❑ Corn
- ❑ Carrots
- ❑ Potatoes (yellow, red, sweet)
- ❑ Red, yellow, orange, or green peppers
- ❑ Butternut, acorn, or summer squash
- ❑ Onions (yellow and green)
- ❑ Mixed greens
- ❑ Garlic (cloves or minced in jar)
- ❑ Tomato (fresh, canned)
- ❑ Tomato paste, tomato sauces

Condiments, sweets and other kitchen staples:

- ☐ Salad dressing
- ☐ Honey
- ☐ Ketchup
- ☐ Mustard (dijon, honey, or yellow)
- ☐ Jam or jelly
- ☐ Syrup (maple, chocolate, butterscotch)
- ☐ Whipped cream
- ☐ Ready-made sauces and marinades
- ☐ Vinegar (balsamic, cider, distilled, rice, or wine)
- ☐ Lemon or lime juice
- ☐ Horseradish
- ☐ Broths (Beef, chicken, vegetable: canned, cubes, granules)
- ☐ Creamed soups (canned)
- ☐ Salsa
- ☐ Soy sauce (low sodium)
- ☐ Baking powder, baking soda
- ☐ Cake mixes
- ☐ Chocolate chips
- ☐ Cornstarch
- ☐ Flour (all-purpose or whole-wheat)
- ☐ Instant pudding and gelatin
- ☐ Hot cocoa packets
- ☐ Sugar (confectioners, granulated, brown)
- ☐ Extracts (vanilla, almond, coconut)

Snack foods

- ❑ Pretzels
- ❑ Crackers (saltines, graham crackers)
- ❑ Chips
- ❑ Sandwich crackers
- ❑ Popcorn
- ❑ Single-serving pudding, custard, gelatin
- ❑ Cereal
- ❑ Ice pops
- ❑ Granola bars
- ❑ Canned fruit
- ❑ Energy bars (Power Bar, ClifBars, Balance Bars, Luna Bars, NuGo bars)

Supplemental powders

- ❑ Carnation Instant Breakfast packets
- ❑ Wheat germ
- ❑ Flax seed powder
- ❑ Non-fat dry milk powder
- ❑ Protein powder (Beneprotein, Unjury)

Liquid supplement drinks

Talk to your dietitian about choosing the right supplement for you; this list names just a few:

- ❑ Ensure Plus, Boost Plus
- ❑ Carnation Instant Breakfast Plus or VHC
- ❑ Boost Glucose Control (Diabetic)
- ❑ Glucerna Shake (Diabetic)

Chapter 7

Life After Treatment

Diet for Cancer Survivors

Now that you've completed active treatment, it's time to move on to the next chapter of your life: survivorship. After finishing treatment, many of you will feel a sense of relief and excitement at having finished such a physically challenging time in your life and grateful to have your life and health. These feelings may go hand-in-hand with feeling afraid, worried, and scared to be on your own without the attention of doctors and nurses, as well as concerned about what happens next in your life. If you are feeling somewhat fearful about your future, this is normal for cancer survivors, and many survivors say that it can take months to feel like your normal self again. Treatment side effects might make it difficult to resume your pre-cancer activities immediately after finishing treatment. Instead of expecting everything to jump right back to normal right after treatment, it is more reasonable to expect a gradual improvement in usual life routines and normalcy. You should allow yourself some time to adjust to changes in your daily routine and diet, so you can recover and feel healthy again.

For most of you, the side effects you experienced during treatment will gradually disappear the longer you've been out of treatment. If you continue to experience some side effects that are still causing weight loss, please continue to follow the list of recommendations for managing side effects and weight loss. You may continue to have symptoms for several weeks or months, such as dry mouth, thick saliva, poor appetite, taste changes, difficulty swallowing, or weight loss. Only when you are feeling almost back to your usual self with your usual appetite, and your weight is stable and within a healthy range (you can discuss this with your healthcare team) should you begin to incorporate healthy eating for cancer survivors. Your doctor or dietitian can help guide you when the time is right for you to change your focus to healthy eating for survivorship.

Now is the time in your life when you should focus on making healthy lifestyle changes. A healthy lifestyle is one that promotes good health and wellness by eating well, exercising, and reducing stress. Research shows that the best way to prevent cancer is proper nutrition along with maintaining a healthy weight and exercise. Some of the major risk factors for cancer are using tobacco products, drinking too much alcohol, being overweight or obese, not eating enough of the healthy nutrients, and getting too much sun exposure without protection. Healthy lifestyle behaviors are important to help prevent the recurrence of cancer, as well as reduce your risk for other chronic diseases, such as heart disease and diabetes. Most people think of "diets" as a life of restrictions. Avoid thinking like this and, instead, think of nourishing your body with the wide range of healthy nutrients found in healthy foods.

Based on the AICR's Second Expert Report, *Food, Nutrition, Physical Activity and the Prevention of Cancer: A Global Perspective* (2007) and the American Cancer Society's (ACS) recommendations for cancer prevention, the following list will help guide you for healthy living after cancer treatment:

1. **Maintain a healthy body weight.** Maintaining a healthy body weight is important for everyone, not only cancer survivors. Having too much fat on your body can increase your risk for many diseases, such as cancer, diabetes, heart disease, hypertension, stroke, and arthritis. Studies have shown that being overweight or obese, or gaining a significant amount of weight during treatment can raise the chances of cancer recurrence. There are two ways we typically measure body fat: Body Mass Index (BMI method) and waist circumference. While neither method is perfect and both methods have some limitations, they do give some insight into your weight status and body fat, if you need to think about losing weight, and if you are at risk for certain diseases.

    BMI: The BMI method is used to determine if a person's weight status is considered *underweight, healthy, overweight, or obese.* BMI is a measure of total body fat based on your height and weight, which is related to your risk of disease and death. You should aim to be within the healthy range for BMI (BMI 18.5 to 24.9). To calculate your BMI:

$$\text{BMI} = \left(\frac{\text{weight in pounds}}{(\text{height in inches}) \times (\text{height in inches})} \right) \times 703$$

For example: A person who weighs 150 pounds, and is 5 feet, 3 inches tall, has a BMI of 26.5

$$\left(\frac{150 \text{ lbs}}{(63 \text{ inches}) \times (63 \text{ inches})} \right) \times 703 = 26.5$$

Your BMI score means the following:

BMI	Weight Status
Below 18.5	Underweight
18.5–24.9	Healthy
25.0–29.9	Overweight
30.0 and above	Obese

You can use the National Heart and Lung Institute's BMI Calculator at *www.nhlbisupport.com/bmi* or Google the words "BMI calculator." Although BMI can be a useful tool for assessment of your overall health status, BMI does have its limitations and, therefore, should be used in conjunction with other data, such as your medical condition, family history, body composition, body fat percentage, and so on. The limitations of BMI are that it may *overestimate* body fat in athletes and those who have a more muscular body, and it may *underestimate* body fat in older persons and those who have lost bone or muscle mass.

Waist Circumference: Checking your waist circumference is another method to assess your body fat. Using a tape measure, place it around your waist right above the tip of your hip bone. Be sure to exhale and then measure your waist. Your waist circumference can determine if you're at health risk. For women, a waist circumference of 31.5 inches or more, and for men, a waist circumference of 37 inches or more indicates high risk.

2. No more excuses—it's time to exercise! Aim to be physically active for at least 30 minutes every day. Being physically active helps prevent cancer, avoid weight gain, strengthen your immune system, aid in digestion and keeping your hormone levels healthy,

reduce stress, and improve your mood. All of those benefits from a half hour a day of breaking a sweat— sounds like a good deal to me! Check with your doctor before starting any exercise program, and always start slowly with moderate activity, such as brisk walking. You can do 30 minutes of moderate exercise at one time or you can do short bouts of activity that total 30 minutes every day (such as 10 minutes x 3 times). Moderate activity is anything that gets your heart beating a little faster and makes you breathe a little deeper. As you progress, health experts recommend that you aim to do at least 60 minutes of moderate activity or 30 minutes of vigorous activity every day. Vigorous activity includes any exercise that raises your heart rate, makes you sweat, and makes you feel out of breath. Some different ideas for physical activity include: walking, hiking, jogging, cycling, swimming or water aerobics, gardening or outdoor work, playing sports you enjoy, dance or movement classes, and breathing exercises. I would suggest, if possible, pairing up with an exercise partner or friend to meet for exercise so you avoid skipping it. Most people are more successful with regular exercise if they schedule it and plan their day around it. Planning ahead prevents you from making excuses.

3. Cut back on sugar and avoid high-calorie foods with little nutritional value. Instead of choosing high-fat and high-sugar foods, aim to include healthy foods and adopt a plant-based diet that includes whole-grains, fruits, vegetables, and beans. Research has found that regularly drinking sugary drinks, such as soda and juices, contributes to weight gain. The biggest problem with sugar-filled drinks is that the calories in these drinks add up very quickly but don't

make you feel full. Choose low-calorie, low-sugar drinks, such as water, sparkling water, unsweetened tea, seltzer, sugar-free flavored waters, and coffee. Avoid highly processed foods and foods with refined sugar. When reading food labels, check the first few ingredients for added sugars such as corn syrup, high-fructose corn syrup, fruit juice concentrate, maltose, dextrose, sucrose, honey, and maple syrup. Although 100-percent fruit juice contains sugar, it is okay in moderation (about one cup per day), as this counts as one of your recommended fruit servings per day.

4. **Adopt a plant-based diet based on the American Institute for Cancer Research's (AICR) "The New American Plate"** (this is available from the AICR by calling 800-843-8114 or accessing it on their Website at *www.aicr.org*). The AICR recommends that we eat most of our foods from plant-based sources. While this does not suggest that you go out and become a strict vegetarian, it does mean that you should try to include most of your daily foods from plant sources. Think of natural foods in their purest forms with the least amount of processing. Eat a variety of vegetables, fruits, whole grains, and legumes, such as beans. There is strong evidence that a mostly plant-based diet cuts down the risk of cancer. Many studies have demonstrated that people who eat diets rich in fruits and vegetables and less meat and animal fats have lower rates of some cancers, such as lung, breast, colon, and stomach cancers. Plant foods contain antioxidants such as beta-carotene, lycopene, and vitamins A, C, and E, as well as phytochemicals that may block the action of carcinogens (cancer-causing substances). Eating a diet that emphasizes plant-based foods is ideal for reducing your risk of cancer, as well as reducing your risk for other diseases.

When making a meal, try to fill two-thirds of your plate with vegetables, fruits, whole grains, and legumes. Not only do these foods provide antioxidants and phytochemicals, but they are also healthy sources of protein, carbohydrates, fat, vitamins, and minerals. Fish, poultry, meat, and low-fat dairy foods should cover no more than one third of the plate. There are thousands of phytochemicals that come in different colored fruits and vegetables, so be sure to include a colorful variety of fruits and vegetables every day.

5. **Limit your intake of red meats (beef, pork, lamb) and avoid processed meats such as ham, bacon, salami, hot dogs, and sausages.** When the term processed is used with meats, it refers to meats that have been smoked, cured, or salted, or contain added preservatives. Studies show that meat-eaters tend to eat less plant-based food, so they are getting less of the protective properties from plant sources. Avoid smoked, cured, or salted meats, as these contain carcinogens (cancer-causing substances), which can damage healthy cells.

6. **Limit your intake of alcoholic drinks to one per day for women and two per day for men.** One drink is equal to 12 ounces of beer, 4 ounces of wine, 1.5 ounces of 80-proof spirits, or 1 ounce of 100-proof spirits. There is evidence that alcohol increases your risk of cancers of the mouth, pharynx, larynx, esophagus, liver, breast, and colon. Moderate amounts (as listed here) can be heart protective; however, more than that increases your risk for cancer. While it may be heart protective to drink red wine for its flavonoid and antioxidant components, the American Heart Association (AHA) recommends that you should not start drinking alcohol to prevent heart disease. The

health benefits that come from red wine come from a phytochemical called *resveratrol,* which you can also find in red and purple grapes, grape juice, raisins, and peanuts; the skin of grapes has the most resveratrol. According to the AICR, red wine is not a recommended source of resveratrol.

7. **Put down the salt shaker.** I used to say that if I could, I would eat salt on top of salt! As a salt lover, I understand how the salt habit can be a hard one to kick. You have to be a little daring and try out alternative spices to get flavor from your foods without adding salt. Just one teaspoon of table salt contains about as much sodium as our daily allowance of sodium—2,400 mg. Foods preserved and processed with salt account for most of our salt intake. Most Americans consume more than the recommended amount of sodium on a daily basis, but there are some things you can do to fix this. Be sure to read Nutrition Facts labels and check the sodium content of foods. Also, avoid foods that are smoked and pickled. Even if something doesn't taste particularly salty, salt can be hidden in cereals, bread, frozen meals, pizza, chips, canned products (soups and sauces), processed meats, and even cookies. When cooking and eating homemade meals, replace salt with new flavors and herbs such as garlic, onions, rosemary, sage, thyme, oregano, celery seed, ginger, cumin, turmeric, caraway, mint, dill, lemongrass, cardamom, fennel, and fenugreek. You can also try Mrs. Dash salt-free seasoning products. Studies have shown that a high salt intake can damage the lining of the stomach, which might increase the risk of stomach cancer (according to the expert panel of the AICR).

8. **To reduce your risk of cancer, don't use supplements and pills.** Choose a balanced diet with a variety of foods. Instead of popping pills, be more thoughtful with what you eat and you will get the nutrients you need from what you eat and drink. Some high dose supplements may actually increase cancer risk. You should make your daily food choices by using the U.S. Department of Agriculture's (USDA) Food Guide Pyramid (2005). You can access it online at *www.my-pyramid.gov*. The pyramid was designed as a guide to healthy, nutritious eating that promotes a healthy diet of adequate nutrients and calories. It is divided into six food groups: grains, fruits, vegetables, dairy, meat and beans, and oils. Similar to the recommendations provided for cancer prevention, it encourages eating whole grains, different colored fruits and vegetables, and lean meats and protein, and limiting fats, sugars, and salt (sodium). Note: there are some situations when supplements are needed, such as women of childbearing age, pregnant women, frail older people, post-menopausal women, and those with known nutrient deficiencies, so talk to your doctor or dietitian for advice. A standard daily multivitamin with minerals that provides 100 percent of the Dietary Reference Intakes (DRIs) may be good for you after treatment, so discuss this with your doctor or dietitian.

9. **If you use currently smoke or tobacco in any form, please ask your doctor about ways to quit.** The research clearly points to the dangers of tobacco and its cause of lung, mouth, throat, pancreas, cervical, and bladder cancers. Dropping the habit can cut your risk for cancer by 30 percent.

Tips for getting started on a healthy lifestyle

- Aim to eat *at least* five servings of a variety of fruits and vegetables per day. I'm sure that many of you have heard of the recommendation for fruits and vegetables: "5-a-Day." What's new about this advice is that some health experts say we should actually get up to nine servings per day of fruits and veggies for the most beneficial health effects! In general, when it comes to fruits and vegetables, the brighter the color, the more nutrients it contains. If you are overweight, choose more vegetables and less fruit, as vegetables contain fewer calories. For example, you can eat four vegetable and three fruit servings. While fresh and frozen are the better ways to eat fruits and vegetables, dried and canned versions also count toward your recommended daily amount. To make this advice meaningful to you, I will explain what an actual serving is and how you can get five to nine servings per day. It's actually not that hard if you pay attention to the portion sizes you are eating. One serving of a fruit or vegetable is: 1/2 cup of fruit, 1 medium piece of fruit (apple, banana, orange), 1/4 cup of dried fruit, 3/4 cup (6 ounces) of 100-percent fruit or vegetable juice, 1 cup of leafy vegetables, or 1/2 cup of cooked or raw vegetables. To plan out your day, this is one of the ways you can visualize it: For breakfast, have at least one serving of fruit; for lunch, have at least two servings of vegetables; for dinner, have another two servings of vegetables; and have another one to three servings of fruits as snacks between meals or as dessert. For some quick and easy ways to snack on veggies instead of fruit, look for pre-washed and pre-cut veggies, such as baby carrots, broccoli florets, celery sticks, and peppers. You can also use frozen fruits and vegetables for greater convenience.

- Think of a rainbow. Choose from a variety of different colored fruits and vegetables, including citrus fruits, dark green or deep yellow vegetables, and colorful berries. Think of choosing fruits and vegetables from a box of crayons—mix different colors on your plate and throughout your day. Some ideas for different colors are: green broccoli, spinach, kale, chard, mustard greens, collard greens, and bok choy; blue and purple blueberries, blackberries, eggplant, and purple cabbage; red tomatoes, strawberries, cherries, red peppers, and raspberries; orange carrots, oranges, and sweet potatoes; white cauliflower, garlic, and onions; and yellow squash, lemons, and yellow peppers.

- Aim to include at least three to five servings per week of cruciferous vegetables (broccoli, cauliflower, cabbage, brussels sprouts, bok choy, and kale), which contains *sulforophane,* one of the the phytochemicals that has shown anti-cancer properties.

- Choose whole grains instead of "enriched" grains. Choose whole-grain breads with at least 2 grams or more of fiber per serving, high-fiber, ready-to-eat cereals with at least 3 to 5 grams or more of fiber per serving, and whole-wheat pastas and brown rice with at least 3 grams or more of fiber per serving. A whole grain means it contains three parts: the bran, the endosperm, and germ. Refined grains are made from the endosperm and the bran and germ are removed. The bran and germ contain all of the fiber and many of the vitamins and minerals found in grains, so choosing whole grains provides you more fiber and nutrients than refined grains. Refined grains that have had key nutrients, such as B vitamins and iron, added back in are called "enriched" grains. White bread and white rice are enriched grains. "Fortified" grains have extra nutrients added to the product, as many cereals on the market do. While enriched and fortified grains do contain key nutrients to prevent deficiencies, they do not have fiber, and we know that fiber is linked to reduced risk of cancer. You should be making half of your grains whole and the other half enriched and fortified grains. Aim to eat at least three servings of whole grain products per day. Some examples of whole grains are wheat, oats, barley, rye, quinoa, buckwheat, bulgur wheat, brown rice, wild rice, sorghum, and popcorn. Tortillas, cereals, breads and pastas can all be made with whole grains. Check food labels for the first ingredient listed and make sure it contains one of these whole grains: stone-ground flour, whole-wheat flour, whole-oat flour, whole-grain corn, whole-grain barley, whole rye flour, and whole ground millet or triticale. Buy whole wheat flour and use it to make pancakes, muffins, cakes, and cookies.

- Legumes and lentils are good sources of plant-based protein. Try to eat legumes at least a few times every week. Some ideas are peas and beans, such as kidney, great northern, pinto, and black beans. Be creative and try adding these foods to soups, salads, chilis, burritos, pasta, and rice. Nuts and seeds are also good sources of protein, but pay attention to portion sizes because these foods are calorie-dense.

- Cut back on unhealthy fats and replace them with healthy fats found in fish, lean meats, poultry, and tofu; olives and olive oil; nuts and seeds; soybeans and soybean oil; vegetable oils such as canola, safflower, sunflower, or flax seed; and vegetable oil margarines. Avoid eating too much saturated fat that comes from animal sources, such as fatty cuts of red meat, cheese, cream, and whole milk. Instead, choose low-fat dairy products such as skim milk, low-fat yogurt, and reduced-fat cheeses, as well as lean meats, such as chicken and turkey. Avoid trans fats found in cookies, cakes, chips, doughnuts, fast food, and other convenience foods. Cut back on added fat in your meals by baking, broiling, or grilling your lean meats, poultry, and fish.

? How can I incorporate a balanced plant-based diet?

Eating a plant-based diet may be very new and different from how you ate before you were diagnosed with cancer. As opposed to the fad diets currently on the market, this type of diet is actually more of a lifestyle change than it is a diet. Start incorporating a healthy, plant-based diet slowly and make small changes every day. Keep telling yourself that eating this way will provide benefits for your long-term health and disease prevention, and help keep you at a healthy weight. However, try to avoid stressing yourself out trying to eat a "perfect" diet. Instead, give yourself time to move toward a lifetime goal of focusing on healthful eating. Take it one day at time and make small, slow changes in your eating patterns. Small, gradual change tends to promote long-lasting habits as opposed to making drastic and unrealistic changes in your eating patterns as seen with many fad diets. Eating nutritiously should help you feel good about yourself—you are nourishing your body with healthy substances to live longer.

? Are there any other tips for maximizing my diet and decreasing my risk for cancer?

- Eat foods that contain vitamin D, such as salmon, sardines, fortified orange juice, milk, reduced-fat cheese, and fortified cereal. Research suggests that vitamin D, which you can also get from sun exposure, may decrease the risk of cancer recurrence. Those who live in a region with limited sun exposure may be deficient (especially in colder months), and people over 50 require more vitamin D, so ask your doctor or dietitian if you should be taking a vitamin D supplement and what dose. You can also have your vitamin D levels checked for a deficiency.

- Eat omega-3 fats, such as salmon, sardines, canned tuna twice a week, and include other sources of omega-3 fats, such as walnuts, flaxseeds, avocados, canola oil, and products fortified with omega-3s.

- Try to eat fermented foods a few times per week, such as yogurt, as these foods contain healthy bacteria called *probiotics*, which improve digestion and immune function, keep your gut healthy, and may prevent cancer.

- Avoid cooking meat, poultry, and fish at very high temperatures, such as cooking over an open flame. Frying, broiling, or grilling meats at very high temperatures may cause cancer-promoting substances to form on the meat. To still enjoy a barbeque once in a while, you can make grilling safer by making some changes, such as marinating the meats in acidic ingredients, such as lemon juice or vinegar mixed with some oil and seasoning. Instead of cooking directly over a flame, cook on a piece of foil. You can also first cook the meat in the oven and then place it on the grill to get some flavor. Avoid eating any meat that is charred or burned. Grilled vegetables and meat-free burgers are another alternative.

- Keep your foods safe by following some of the food safety guidelines discussed in Chapter 1 of this book, such as washing your hands, counters, dishes, cutting board, and utensils well; avoiding cross-contamination of raw meat, fish, or poultry; thawing frozen foods in the microwave or refrigerator; using a food thermometer to check that your meat is fully cooked;

and always checking the expiration dates on food and throwing out foods if you think they might be spoiled.

I think that by now you can see that healthy living for disease prevention—ranging from cancer to heart disease to diabetes—one that involves a healthy diet of plant-based foods, physical activity, and maintaining a healthy body weight.

Chapter 8

Nutrition and Cancer Resources

When you Google the words "cancer and nutrition," you find more than 58 million results. When you Google the words "nutrition and cancer," you find more than 39 million results, and when you Google the words "vitamins and minerals and cancer," you find more than 1 million results (accessed January 2010). Needless to say, there is a lot of information accessible on the Internet, some coming from reliable and credible sources, and some that is not. Use caution and common sense, and stay alert when reading anything on the Internet or in a magazine or hearing a news report. Avoid any products that claim to cure disease or promise a miracle. Pills, powders, and other products are often marketed to cancer survivors with unverified health claims not based on scientific evidence. You can talk to your doctor or dietitian if you are looking for more information from reputable sources. As always, talk to him or her before starting any new strategy, diet, or supplement you read or hear about from the news, magazines, or the Internet.

How do I navigate through the plethora of information available on the Internet?

- When looking at the source, check to see if it's a credible source, such as a health organization or government Website, such as *www.mypyramid.gov* or *www. nih.gov*.

- Be wary of information coming from a supplement manufacturer or someone recommending taking lots of supplement pills. Many supplements are not tested for effectiveness and safety.

- When searching the Web, you can also check the URL, such as .gov (government Website), .edu (educational Website), and .org (nonprofit organization).

- When reading Websites, check the credentials of the author, if academic journals are referenced in the article, and the date the site was last updated.

- Verify anything you read on the Internet or hear in the news with your doctor or dietitian.

 How can I spot diet quackery?

- Promises a quick fix with fast weight loss, disease prevention, or a medical miracle.

- Uses words like "breakthrough," "miracle," "discovery," "magic bullet" and "quick fix."

- Bans certain food or groups of food; often promotes unbalanced nutrient intake.

- Based on flawed or biased research study; based on a single study.

- Helps to sell a product or supplement.

- Suggests that a certain food can change your body chemistry.
- Diet based on one main food or supplement.

? What are some signs of a scam?

According to the Federal Trade Commission, there are some warning signs that you can look for in an ad or Website to see if it's a scam:

- Any Website or claim that says it can treat everyone with cancer.
- Just because a product says it's "natural" doesn't mean it's effective or safe for treating cancer, and it can even be harmful. Scammers often promote unproven and potentially dangerous remedies for treating cancer.
- They market personal stories, "case histories," and "testimonials" about the product; however, these stories can be completely fake, and the people may have been paid to endorse the product. Personal stories are not reliable sources as conclusive evidence of effectiveness.
- They use medical jargon and fancy words, but this is not the same as hearing it straight from your doctor.
- If they state there is a money-back guarantee, this does not mean that the product is effective or safe.

? Who is considered a nutrition expert?

Many people call themselves nutrition experts or nutritionists without meeting the requirements of Registered Dietitians (RD). The initials RD mean that the person has met the educational and experience requirements by the American Dietetic

Association to attain the title, which includes a bachelor's degree, completion of a Commission on Accreditation for Dietetics Education (CADE) program and a dietetic internship, passing a standardized national exam, and completing continuing education credits to maintain the title. RDs can refer to themselves as a "nutritionist" or "dietitian," but not all nutritionists are dietitians and anyone can call him- or herself a "nutritionist." Because "nutritionist" is not usually a licensed title, be sure to check if the person has the appropriate credentials (the letters RD after someone's name). You can also access a nutritional professional by going to the American Dietetic Association's Website: *www.eatright.org*. There are also licensed nutritionists, such as Certified Nutrition Specialist (CNS), the license for which does not require intensive hands-on clinical experience, and Certified Dietetic Nutritionist (CDN) which requires clinical experience.

? Can you give me a list of reliable resources for information on nutrition and cancer?

- **Caring 4 Cancer:** *www.caring4cancer.com/go/cancer/nutrition*
- **American Institute for Cancer Research (AICR):** *www.aicr.org*; 1-800-843-8114.
- **American Cancer Society (ACS):** *www.cancer.org*
- **National Cancer Institute (NCI):** *www.cancer.gov*
- **Medline Plus:** *www.nlm.nih.gov/medlineplus*
- **Oncology Nutrition; Dietetic Practice Group of The American Dietetic Association:** *www.oncology-nutrition.org*
- **CURE Magazine:** *http://curetoday.com*
- **Guide To Internet Resources for Cancer:** *http://cancerindex.org*

- **Food and Drug Administration:** *http://www.fda.gov*
- **American Dietetic Association:** *www.eatright.org* You can find a list of registered dietitians or can call the Nutrition Information Hotline: 1-800-366-1655.
- **Food and Nutrition Information Center (FNIC), National Agriculture Library;** U.S. Department of Agriculture: *www.nal.usda.gov/fnic*
- **Diana Dyer's Website:** *http://cancerRD.com*
- **U.S. Department of Health and Human Services, Health Finder:** *www.healthfinder.gov*
- **National Coalition for Cancer Survivorship:** *www.cansearch.org*

? Can you list reliable resources for finding information on complementary practices?

- **Memorial Sloan-Kettering Cancer Center Integrative Medicine:** *www.mskcc.org/mskcc/html/11570.cfm?herbsac* and *www.mskcc.org/mskcc/html/11917.cfm*
- **National Center for Complementary and Alternative Medicine of the National Institutes for Health:** *http://nccam.nih.gov/health/*
- **Medline Plus:** *www.nlm.nih.gov/medlineplus/druginfo/herb_All.html#A*
- **NIH, Office of Dietary Supplements:** *http://ods.od.nih.gov/Health_Information/Health_Information.aspx*
- **Consumer Lab:** *www.consumerlab.com*
- **Office of Dietary Supplements: National Cancer Institute:** *www.cancer.gov/cam*

- **FDA Center For Food Safety and Applied Nutrition: Dietary Supplements:** *www.cfsan.fda.gov/~dms/ds-savvy.html www.cfsan.fda.gov/~dms/ds-warn.html*

- **FDA MedWatch:** *www.fda.gov/medwatch/index.html*

- **Natural Standard Database:** *www.naturalstandard.com*

? Can you list some reliable sources for more information on Food Safety Recommendations?

- **American Cancer Society, food handling tips:** *www.cancer.org/docroot/MBC/content/MBC_6_2X_Food_Handling_Tips.asp?sitearea=MBC*

- **Fred Hutchinson Cancer Research Center:** *www.fhcrc.org/science/clinical/ltfu/patient/food_safety_guidelines.pdf* Patients undergoing a stem cell transplant can also read the following "Guidelines for Immunosuppressed Patients:" *www.fhcrc.org/science/clinical/ltfu/patient/diet_guidelines.html*

- **FDA Center for Food Safety and Applied Nutrition**: *www.cfsan.fda.gov*

Chapter 9

Debunking Myths: Frequently Asked Questions About Nutrition and Cancer

With so much information out there about nutrition and cancer, it's difficult to decipher what is fact and what is fiction. Aside from information you may hear on the news or read on the Internet, you may also hear anecdotal or word-of-mouth reports about diet and cancer. I hear it over and over from my patients, "My friend's sister's husband knew someone who told him to eat...." The following questions address hot topics and common questions I hear from patients on a daily basis.

? I've heard that there is a connection between sugar and cancer and that I should avoid eating sugar. Is it true that sugar "feeds" cancer?

No. The research has not shown sugar to directly increase the risk of causing cancer. However, it's a good idea to limit the amount of simple sugars you eat, which add a lot of calories without providing cancer-preventive nutrients and can cause weight gain and obesity, which is linked to an increased cancer risk.

This doesn't mean you can never touch any dessert or sugary food ever again; it just means you need to keep the word "moderation" in mind when it comes to sweets. Limit the amount of simple sugars you eat, which is found in honey, raw sugar, brown sugar, corn syrup, and molasses, as well as sugary drinks such as soda and fruit-flavored drinks. Limit your intake of cakes, cookies, candy, and sugar cereals. The best way to eat sugar or carbohydrates is *along with* protein, fat, and fiber. These foods help your body optimally process the sugar at a slower pace. For example, have a piece of fruit with a few tablespoons of peanut butter or nuts. The peanut butter and nuts contain fat, protein, and fiber, which help balance the sugar in the fruit. You should also choose carbohydrates that naturally contain fiber, such as whole-wheat bread and fruit. When it comes to sugar and carbohydrates, your best bet (when you have finished treatment) is choosing most often naturally occurring sugar like the sugar found in fruit (fructose) and milk (lactose). Keep an eye on portion sizes, be mindful to indulge in these treats only a few times per week, and aim to eat healthy, unprocessed foods such as fruit, vegetables, whole grains, legumes, nuts and seeds.

? Are organic foods better than non-organic (conventional) foods for people with cancer?

The term organic refers to plant foods grown without pesticides, herbicides, and genetic modifications, and meats, poultry, eggs and dairy products that come from animals that have not been given antibiotics or growth hormones. There is conflicting information about this topic, so it's confusing to decide what is best to do. Some suggest that eating organic foods is healthier because it reduces your exposure to chemicals and pesticides. Some studies have shown that organic fruits and vegetables contain higher amounts of healthy nutrients and vitamins. On the other side, some argue that organic foods spoil faster and are more susceptible to contamination by insects, mold, and fungus. However, recent studies suggest that organic food is just as safe as non-organic food. There is no research in humans that shows that organic foods are better for reducing the risk, recurrence, or progression of cancer, and there are no good studies showing that the trace amounts of pesticides found on fruits and vegetables are linked with cancer or other diseases. However, we do know that those people exposed to large amounts of pesticides and chemicals can have an increased risk of cancer. For this reason, some people choose to eat organic fruits and vegetables to keep our planet and community as healthy as possible.

If you wish to limit your exposure to pesticides, you should choose organic fruits and vegetables when possible; however, if it is difficult for you to afford or find organic foods, you should not avoid eating non-organic fruits and vegetables out of fear of pesticides. The research is clear about one thing: eating more fruits and vegetables (whether organic or not) lowers your risk of cancer and other diseases. You will always receive the cancer-protective effects of eating fruits and vegetables whether they are organic or conventionally grown. Always aim to eat five or more servings per day of fruits and vegetables, no matter how they are grown.

If you would like to reduce your exposure to pesticides found on fruits and vegetables, the Environmental Working Group helps guide consumers when selecting fruits and vegetables by giving two lists: "the dirty dozen" (most chemical residues) and the "the clean fifteen" (the least chemical residues). "The dirty dozen" includes: peaches, apples, nectarines, strawberries, cherries, grapes (imported), pears, sweet bell peppers, celery, kale, lettuce, and carrots. "The clean fifteen" includes: onions, avocados, sweet corn, pineapples, mangoes, asparagus, sweet peas, kiwis, cabbage, eggplant, papayas, watermelon, broccoli, tomatoes, and sweet potatoes.

When it comes to processed foods, such as crackers, cakes, and cookies, instead of worrying about whether the product is organic, you should focus on choosing those made with whole grains, that are low in sugar and saturated fats, and are trans-fat free. Don't be fooled into thinking that just because a product is listed as "organic" means that it's healthy for you. Organic sugar and non-organic sugar contain the same amount of calories and both can cause weight gain when eaten in excess. An organic cupcake with frosting is no better for you than a non-organic cupcake with frosting. As for meat and dairy products, it is more important to focus on eating low-fat and lean animal products to limit your daily saturated and total fat, and to make sure you are eating appropriate portion sizes.

? Is there anything I should avoid eating that may interact with my treatment?

The only times you need to avoid eating foods that interact with treatment are: if you are on a medication that interacts with a specific food, vitamin, or mineral; if you are experiencing a side effect from treatment that requires you to avoid certain foods to alleviate the symptom; or you have had surgery. Otherwise, you do not need to avoid any special foods. Your healthcare team will tell you if you need to avoid a food or nutrient because of a medication or treatment. You should avoid taking any supplements during treatment that contain high dose antioxidants (more than 100 percent of the Dietary Reference Intakes [DRIs]), such as vitamins C and E, beta-carotene, and selenium. You should also talk to your healthcare team about starting any herbal supplements such as supplementing with garlic, ginkgo, echinacea, soy supplements, ginseng, St. John's Wort, valerian, kava, and grape seed as some may potentially interact with a medication or treatment.

? Should I be taking vitamins and minerals during treatment?

You should only be taking vitamins and minerals if you are told to do so by your healthcare team. If you are underweight, elderly, or not eating well, you may need to take a standard daily multivitamin and mineral supplement that contains about 100 percent of the DRIs for most nutrients during treatment. You should be cautious about taking high-dose vitamins, minerals, or other supplements because they may interfere with treatment. There are situations in which single vitamins or minerals, such as vitamins B12 or D, calcium, or iron are prescribed by your physician for a diagnosed deficiency or medical condition. Only supplement with single nutrients if you have cleared it with your healthcare team.

If you are cleared to take a dietary supplement, you can choose the product by checking to see if the label has a USP Verified Mark, which means that the product has been verified by the USP Dietary Supplement Verification Program (a nonprofit, federally recognized organization that offers voluntary testing and establishes standards of quality for medications and dietary supplements). The USP Mark ensures the quality, purity, and potency of the dietary supplement. You can see a list of USP Verified Dietary Supplements on www.*usp.org/USPVerified/dietarySupplements/supplements.html*. You can also check *www.consumerlab.com* for reputable dietary supplements that have been tested for quality and purity.

? Should I be drinking more juice to meet the recommendations for fruits and vegetables?

While juices can provide important nutrients, including vitamin C, beta-carotene, and potassium, as well as other antioxidants that reduce the risk of major diseases, such as heart disease and cancer, they do provide less fiber and antioxidants found in the peels and skins of fruits and vegetables. Additionally, juices are much less filling and contain more concentrated amounts of calories than eating the actual fruit or vegetable in its whole form, which means drinking juice makes it is easier to consume excess calories and gain weight. Studies show that people do not make up for calories they drink by eating less food, yet people do feel fuller and eat fewer calories when eating high-fiber foods, such as fruits and vegetables. If you drink juices to meet your daily needs for fruits and vegetables, be sure to drink in moderation—about one or two servings (one serving = 6 ounces) per day. When buying commercial juices, they should be pasteurized and 100-percent fruit or vegetable juices. If you are having difficulty chewing or swallowing during or after treatment, you should be including juices every day to help obtain essential nutrients.

? Do artificial sweeteners, like saccharin and aspartame, cause cancer?

No, the evidence thus far does not show any link between these sweeteners and increased cancer risk. Saccharin used to be thought of as a carcinogen because of studies on rats, but it has not been shown to cause cancer in humans, so it has been removed from the lists of carcinogens by the U.S. National Toxicology Program.

Index

About the Author

Jodi Buckman Weinstein, MS, RD, CSO, CDN is a registered dietitian, board certified specialist in oncology nutrition, and certified dietitian-nutritionist in New York City. She received a master's degree in nutrition and dietetics from New York University. Jodi currently is the clinical nutrition coordinator at the Tisch Cancer Institute at Mount Sinai Medical Center. She also leads a comprehensive weight management group class and maintains a private nutrition counseling practice, in which she provides individualized counseling to adults dealing with a variety of nutritional concerns. Jodi has facilitated community workshops and lectures on healthy eating and wellness, contributed nutrition articles to various newsletters, led cancer support groups, been interviewed as a nutrition expert for television and newspapers, participated in nutrition research studies, and lectured to physicians and nurses at conferences, as well as to people living with diseases, such as cancer and multiple sclerosis. Jodi is a member of the American Dietetic Association, the New York State Dietetic Association, and the Dietitians in Oncology Nutrition Practice Group. Jodi was recently married in her hometown of Chicago, Illinois, and is living with her husband in New York City.

Books of Similar Interest

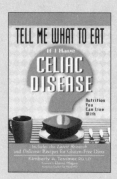

Tell Me What to Eat If I Have Celiac Disease
Nutrition You Can Live With

EAN 978-1-60163-061-2
U.S. $12.99

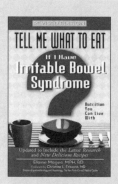

Tell Me What to Eat If I Have Irritable Bowel Syndrome
Nutrition You Can Live With

EAN 978-1-60163-021-6
U.S.$12.99

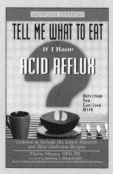

Tell Me What to Eat If I Have Acid Reflux
Nutrition You Can Live With

EAN 978-1-60163-019-3
U.S. $12.99

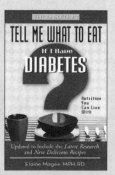

Tell Me What to Eat If I Have Diabetes
Nutrition You Can Live With

EAN 978-1-60163-021-6
U.S. $12.99

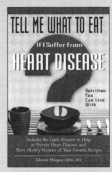
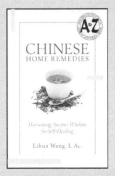
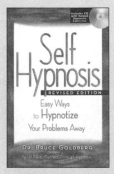